Diverticulitis CookBook

Dietary Guide with Safe Recipes to improve Gut Health

William Moritz

Copyright

No part of this book should be copied, reproduced without the author's permission © 2024

TABLE OF CONTENT

Part I. Understanding Diverticular Disease

Introducing Diverticulosis and Diverticulitis

Diverticulosis and diverticulitis are common gastrointestinal conditions that primarily affect the large intestine, or colon. Understanding the basics of these conditions is essential for individuals seeking to manage their digestive health effectively.

Diverticulosis:

Diverticulosis is characterized by the presence of small pouches, known as diverticula, that form along the walls of the colon. These pouches develop when weak spots in the colon's muscle layers allow the inner lining to bulge outward. While diverticulosis itself typically does not cause noticeable symptoms, it is often discovered incidentally during diagnostic tests such as colonoscopy or imaging studies. The prevalence of diverticulosis increases with age, and it is more commonly observed in industrialized nations where low-fiber diets are prevalent. While the exact cause of diverticulosis is not fully understood, factors such as age, genetics, and dietary choices are believed to contribute to its development.

Diverticulitis:
Diverticulitis occurs when diverticula become inflamed or infected. This condition can lead to a range of symptoms, including abdominal pain, fever, nausea, and changes in bowel habits. Complications may arise if the inflammation causes the formation of abscesses, perforations, or other severe conditions. Unlike diverticulosis, diverticulitis often requires medical attention and intervention. Diagnosis is typically based on a combination of medical history, physical examination, and diagnostic tests such as CT scans.

Connection Between Diverticulosis and Diverticulitis:
While diverticulosis itself may be asymptomatic, understanding its presence is crucial as it can potentially progress to diverticulitis. Managing diverticulosis involves adopting a healthy lifestyle, including a high-fiber diet, to prevent inflammation and complications. Individuals diagnosed with diverticulitis may require antibiotics, dietary modifications, and, in severe cases, surgical intervention. Overall, an awareness of both diverticulosis and diverticulitis empowers individuals to take proactive steps towards maintaining a healthy digestive system and preventing the progression of these conditions.

Importance of Digestive Health

Digestive health is of paramount importance as it directly influences overall well-being and quality of life. The digestive system is intricately linked to the body's ability to absorb essential nutrients, maintain a healthy immune system, and eliminate waste efficiently. Optimal digestive health ensures that the body receives the necessary nutrients for energy production, tissue repair, and proper functioning of organs.

An efficient digestive system contributes to immune resilience, as a significant portion of the immune system is housed in the gastrointestinal tract. A well-balanced gut microbiome, consisting of beneficial bacteria, plays a crucial role in protecting against infections and supporting immune responses.

Beyond physical health, digestive well-being influences mental and emotional states. The gut-brain connection highlights how the health of the digestive system can impact mood, stress levels, and cognitive function. A harmonious gut environment is associated with reduced instances of mood disorders and improved mental clarity.

In the context of diverticulosis and diverticulitis, understanding and maintaining digestive health become even more critical. Promoting a balanced and fiber-rich diet, staying hydrated, exercising regularly, and managing stress are key components of preserving digestive health. Recognizing the importance of digestive well-being empowers individuals to make informed lifestyle choices, fostering a holistic approach to health and preventing the onset or progression of gastrointestinal conditions.

Scope and Objectives of the Book

The scope and objectives of this comprehensive book on diverticulosis and diverticulitis are designed to cater to a diverse audience, ranging from individuals seeking preventive measures to those grappling with the challenges of managing these gastrointestinal conditions.

Scope:

1. Education for All Audiences:
   - The book aims to be accessible to a broad readership, from those unfamiliar with diverticular diseases to individuals already affected. It serves as a go-to resource for understanding the nuances of diverticulosis and diverticulitis.

2. In-Depth Exploration:

   - Delving into the intricacies of digestive health, the book covers topics such as the anatomy of the digestive system, causes and risk factors, symptom identification, diagnostic procedures, and various treatment options. It offers a comprehensive understanding of these conditions.

3. Practical Guidance:

   - Focused on empowering readers, the book provides practical tips on dietary modifications, lifestyle changes, and long-term management strategies. It seeks to bridge the gap between medical knowledge and actionable steps for readers to incorporate into their daily lives.

Objectives:

1. Awareness and Prevention:

   - To raise awareness about diverticulosis and diverticulitis, emphasizing the importance of preventive measures, early detection, and the adoption of a healthy lifestyle.

2. Comprehensive Guidance:

   - To offer a thorough guide for individuals diagnosed with diverticulosis or diverticulitis, providing them with insights into effective management strategies, treatment options, and long-term well-being.

3. Empowerment Through Knowledge:
  - To empower readers with knowledge, enabling them to make informed decisions about their digestive health. The book seeks to demystify medical concepts, making the information accessible and relatable.

4. Support and Encouragement:
  - To provide a supportive framework through patient testimonials, success stories, and resources, fostering a sense of community and encouragement for those navigating the challenges of diverticular diseases.

In essence, the book aspires to be a comprehensive, informative, and supportive guide that equips readers with the tools they need to understand, manage, and proactively address diverticulosis and diverticulitis for a healthier, more fulfilling life.

CHAPTER ONE

Anatomy of the Digestive System

The anatomy of the digestive system is a marvel of intricate structures and coordinated functions that work together to break down food, absorb nutrients, and eliminate waste. This highly specialized system ensures the body receives the essential elements it needs for energy production, growth, and overall well-being.

1. Mouth and Salivary Glands:
   - The digestive process begins in the mouth, where mechanical digestion commences through chewing, and chemical digestion is initiated by saliva. Salivary glands release enzymes like amylase, which break down complex carbohydrates into simpler sugars.

2. Esophagus:
   - The swallowed food travels down the esophagus, a muscular tube connecting the mouth to the stomach.

Muscular contractions, known as peristalsis, propel the food forward.

3. Stomach:
   - The stomach serves as a reservoir and a site for further digestion. Gastric juices, including hydrochloric acid and digestive enzymes, break down proteins, forming a semi-liquid mixture called chyme.

4. Small Intestine:
   - The majority of nutrient absorption occurs in the small intestine. Divided into the duodenum, jejunum, and ileum, the small intestine receives bile from the liver and pancreatic enzymes, facilitating the breakdown of fats, proteins, and carbohydrates.

5. Liver and Gallbladder:
   - The liver produces bile, crucial for fat digestion, while the gallbladder stores and releases bile into the small intestine as needed.

6. Pancreas:
   - The pancreas secretes digestive enzymes into the small intestine, contributing to the breakdown of nutrients. It also produces insulin and glucagon, regulating blood sugar levels.

7. Large Intestine (Colon):

- The remaining indigestible material moves into the large intestine, where water is absorbed, and the formation of feces occurs. The colon houses a diverse population of bacteria crucial for fermentation and further nutrient absorption.

8. Rectum and Anus:
   - The final stages of digestion take place in the rectum, where feces are stored until elimination through the anus. Muscular contractions, known as peristaltic movements, facilitate the expulsion of waste.

The seamless coordination of these anatomical components ensures the efficiency of the digestive process. Understanding the anatomy of the digestive system is essential for comprehending how various factors, such as diet, lifestyle, and medical conditions, can impact its functioning and, consequently, overall health.

Explanation of the colon and its function

The colon, also known as the large intestine, is a crucial component of the digestive system with distinctive functions vital for nutrient absorption, water reabsorption, and waste elimination. Located between the small intestine and the rectum, the colon plays a central role in the final stages of digestion.

Structure of the Colon:
   - The colon is a tube-like structure, approximately 5 to 6 feet long, and is divided into several segments: the ascending colon, transverse colon, descending colon, and sigmoid colon. It terminates in the rectum, which connects to the anus.

Functions of the Colon:

1. Absorption of Water and Electrolytes:
   - As undigested food material, now referred to as chyme, enters the colon, its liquid consistency is gradually transformed into a more solid form through the absorption of water and electrolytes. This process is crucial for maintaining proper hydration levels in the body.

2. Fermentation and Nutrient Production:
   - The colon houses a vast community of beneficial bacteria, known as the gut microbiota. These microbes play a vital role in fermenting undigested carbohydrates, producing short-chain fatty acids (SCFAs), and synthesizing certain vitamins, such as B vitamins and vitamin K.

3. Formation of Feces:

- As the chyme progresses through the colon, water absorption continues, and the remaining indigestible material forms solid feces. The consistency and composition of feces are influenced by factors such as diet, gut microbiota, and transit time through the colon.

4. Storage and Controlled Elimination:
- The rectum, the final portion of the colon, serves as a storage reservoir for feces until it is ready for elimination. The anal sphincters, muscles surrounding the anus, regulate the controlled release of feces during bowel movements.

Impact on Overall Health:
- The health of the colon is closely linked to overall well-being. A well-functioning colon contributes to regular bowel movements, nutrient absorption, and a balanced gut microbiome. Conversely, issues such as constipation, diarrhea, or inflammation can indicate underlying digestive concerns.

Understanding the structure and functions of the colon is crucial for maintaining digestive health. A diet rich in fiber, hydration, and a balanced microbiome contribute to optimal colon function, supporting overall digestive well-being and systemic health. Regular medical check-ups and screenings are also essential for detecting and addressing any potential issues in a timely manner.

Role of the intestines in digestion

The intestines play a vital role in the digestive process, encompassing both the small and large intestines. Their functions are essential for breaking down food, absorbing nutrients, and facilitating the elimination of waste.

1. Small Intestine:
   - The small intestine is a central player in digestion and nutrient absorption. Comprising the duodenum, jejunum, and ileum, it receives partially digested food from the stomach. Enzymes produced by the pancreas and bile from the liver aid in breaking down proteins, fats, and carbohydrates. The small intestine's extensive surface area, characterized by villi and microvilli, enhances nutrient absorption into the bloodstream.

2. Large Intestine (Colon):
   - The large intestine, or colon, follows the small intestine in the digestive tract. Its primary functions involve absorbing water and electrolytes from the remaining indigestible material, forming feces. The colon houses a diverse population of beneficial

bacteria, contributing to the fermentation of undigested carbohydrates and the production of short-chain fatty acids. While the small intestine focuses on nutrient absorption, the colon ensures efficient water reabsorption and the formation of solid waste.

3. Overall Digestive Coordination:
   - The coordination between the small and large intestines is essential for maintaining digestive health. The small intestine breaks down complex food components into absorbable nutrients, while the colon ensures the regulation of water content and the formation of feces for elimination.

4. Gut Microbiota:
   - Both sections of the intestines host a complex ecosystem of microorganisms collectively known as the gut microbiota. This microbial community aids in digestion, synthesizes certain vitamins, and supports overall gut health. An imbalance in the gut microbiota can lead to digestive issues and impact overall well-being.

Understanding the intricate roles of the small and large intestines in digestion underscores the importance of maintaining their optimal function. A well-balanced diet, sufficient hydration, and a healthy gut microbiome contribute to the seamless operation of these digestive organs, fostering overall digestive efficiency and well-being.

CHAPTER TWO

How Diverticula Form

Diverticula, small pouches that form along the walls of the colon, result from a process known as diverticulosis. This condition arises when weak points in the muscular layers of the colon allow the inner lining to protrude outward, forming these pouch-like structures. The exact mechanisms behind how diverticula form are multifaceted.

The primary contributing factor is believed to be increased pressure within the colon, often associated with a low-fiber diet. A diet lacking in sufficient fiber can lead to constipation and harder stools, requiring more force during bowel movements. This increased pressure over time creates weak spots, particularly at sites where blood vessels penetrate the colon's muscle layers.

As the pressure continues, the inner lining of the colon bulges through these weak areas, forming diverticula. The most common locations for diverticula are in the sigmoid colon, the lower part of the large intestine. While age is a contributing factor, and the prevalence of diverticulosis increases with advancing age, dietary choices and lifestyle factors play a significant role in its development.

Understanding how diverticula form underscores the importance of dietary habits in preventing their onset. A diet rich in fiber helps maintain regular bowel movements, reduces pressure within the colon, and supports overall colon health. By addressing these modifiable factors, individuals can take proactive steps to minimize the risk of diverticulosis and its potential complications.

Weak Areas of the Colon

The formation of diverticula in the colon is closely tied to weak areas within the muscular layers of this digestive organ. These weak areas are commonly found at points where blood vessels penetrate the colon wall. The colon, being a muscular tube responsible for the absorption of water and electrolytes, can experience areas of structural vulnerability, particularly if subjected to increased pressure over time.

The most susceptible region for the development of weak areas is the sigmoid colon, which is the S-shaped segment located at the end of the large intestine. This region is predisposed to heightened pressure due to its anatomical position and the nature of its function in storing and expelling feces.

Weak areas can be exacerbated by factors such as age, genetic predispositions, and lifestyle choices, particularly a low-fiber diet. A diet lacking in sufficient fiber can result in constipation, leading to increased pressure during bowel movements and straining of the colon walls.

Understanding the locations and factors contributing to weak areas in the colon is crucial in comprehending the development of diverticula. By addressing modifiable risk factors like dietary habits and lifestyle choices, individuals can take preventive measures to minimize the likelihood of diverticulosis and promote a healthier digestive system.

Factors Leading to Diverticulosis

Diverticulosis, the condition characterized by the formation of diverticula in the colon, is influenced by a combination of factors, both genetic and lifestyle-related. Understanding these factors is crucial for preventing and managing the development of diverticula.

1. Age: Diverticulosis becomes more prevalent with age, particularly affecting individuals over the age of 50. The aging process may contribute to changes in the structure and function of the colon, making it more susceptible to the formation of diverticula.

2. Genetics: There is evidence to suggest a genetic predisposition to diverticulosis. Individuals with a family history of the condition may be at a higher risk of developing diverticula. Genetic factors can influence the strength and resilience of the colon walls.

3. Dietary Choices: A low-fiber diet is a significant contributor to diverticulosis. Insufficient fiber intake results in constipation, leading to increased pressure in the colon during bowel movements. This heightened pressure can create weak areas in the colon walls, making the formation of diverticula more likely.

4. Lifestyle Factors: Sedentary lifestyles and a lack of regular physical activity may contribute to the development of diverticulosis. Exercise helps maintain healthy bowel function and reduces the risk of constipation, thereby lowering the pressure within the colon.

5. Obesity: Being overweight or obese is associated with an increased risk of diverticulosis. Excess weight can contribute to elevated pressure in the colon, creating conditions conducive to the formation of diverticula.

Addressing these factors through lifestyle modifications, including a high-fiber diet, regular exercise, and maintaining a healthy weight, can significantly reduce the risk of diverticulosis and promote overall digestive health.

CHAPTER THREE

Causes and Risk Factors

The development of diverticulosis and diverticulitis is influenced by a variety of causes and risk factors, ranging from age-related changes to lifestyle choices and genetic predispositions.

1. Age: Aging is a significant factor in the development of diverticulosis. As individuals grow older, the walls of the colon may weaken, making the formation of diverticula more likely. This condition is particularly common in individuals over the age of 50.

2. Genetics: There is evidence to suggest a genetic component to diverticular diseases. Individuals with a family history of diverticulosis may have a higher predisposition to developing these conditions, indicating a potential genetic link.

3. Lifestyle Factors: Dietary choices play a crucial role in diverticulosis. A low-fiber diet, common in many Western societies, can contribute to constipation and increased pressure within the colon, promoting the formation of diverticula. Lack of exercise and sedentary lifestyles also heighten the risk.

4. Obesity: Being overweight or obese is associated with an increased risk of diverticulosis. Excess body weight may contribute to elevated pressure in the colon, facilitating the development of diverticula.

5. Smoking and Lack of Physical Activity: Both smoking and a sedentary lifestyle have been identified as risk factors for diverticulosis. Smoking can adversely affect the blood supply to the colon, while physical inactivity contributes to poor bowel function.

6. Previous Gastrointestinal Conditions: Conditions such as inflammatory bowel disease (IBD) and irritable bowel syndrome (IBS) may increase the likelihood of diverticular diseases.

Understanding these causes and risk factors is crucial for implementing preventive strategies. Adopting a high-fiber diet, engaging in regular physical activity, maintaining a healthy weight, and considering genetic factors during medical assessments are essential steps in reducing the risk of diverticulosis and diverticulitis.

Age and Diverticulosis

Age is a significant factor influencing the development of diverticulosis, a condition characterized by the presence of diverticula (small pouches) in the colon. While diverticulosis can affect individuals of any age, it becomes more prevalent as people grow older, particularly after the age of 50.

As the body ages, the structural and functional changes in the colon contribute to an increased susceptibility to diverticula formation. The natural wear and tear on the digestive system, combined with a gradual loss of muscle tone in the colon, make it more prone to the development of weak areas where diverticula can occur.

The risk of diverticulosis tends to rise with advancing age, reaching a peak in the later decades of life. By the age of 80, a significant portion of the population may have diverticula, though not all individuals will experience symptoms.

While age is a non-modifiable risk factor, understanding its association with diverticulosis underscores the importance of adopting preventive measures earlier in life. Lifestyle choices, including a high-fiber diet, regular physical activity, and maintaining a healthy weight, can mitigate the impact of age on the development of diverticulosis and promote overall digestive well-being.

Relationship between Age and Risk

The relationship between age and the risk of developing diverticulosis is a well-established aspect of this gastrointestinal condition. Diverticulosis, characterized by the presence of small pouches (diverticula) in the colon, becomes more prevalent with advancing age.

As individuals age, structural changes occur in the colon, making it more susceptible to the formation of diverticula. The natural wear and tear on the muscular layers of the colon, combined with a gradual reduction in muscle tone, contribute to the weakening of the colon walls. This weakened state creates areas of vulnerability, particularly in the sigmoid colon, where diverticula often form.

The risk of diverticulosis increases notably after the age of 50, and the likelihood continues to rise with each subsequent decade. By the age of 80, a substantial portion of the population may have diverticula, although not all individuals will experience symptoms or complications.

While age is a non-modifiable risk factor, understanding this relationship emphasizes the importance of proactive measures to promote digestive health in later years. Adopting a diet rich in fiber, maintaining a healthy lifestyle, and seeking regular medical check-ups are crucial steps in managing the age-associated risk of diverticulosis.

Genetics and Diverticular Diseases

Genetics plays a notable role in the development of diverticular diseases, encompassing both diverticulosis and its more severe counterpart, diverticulitis. While lifestyle factors such as diet and exercise are significant contributors, a familial predisposition can heighten an individual's susceptibility to these gastrointestinal conditions.

Genetic Predisposition:
Research suggests a hereditary component in the risk of diverticular diseases. Individuals with a family history of diverticulosis or diverticulitis are more likely to develop these conditions themselves. This familial

clustering suggests a potential genetic link that influences the structural integrity of the colon and its susceptibility to diverticula formation.

Influence on Colon Structure:
Genetic factors may impact the strength and resilience of the colon walls. Variations in the genes associated with the connective tissues and muscular layers of the colon could contribute to an increased likelihood of developing weak areas where diverticula can form. Understanding the specific genetic markers and pathways involved is an ongoing area of research in gastroenterology.

Interplay with Lifestyle Factors:
It's important to note that while genetics can influence susceptibility, lifestyle factors, particularly dietary choices, play a crucial role in the manifestation of diverticular diseases. A diet low in fiber, common in Western societies, can exacerbate the genetic predisposition by promoting constipation and increased pressure in the colon.

Preventive Measures:
Individuals with a family history of diverticular diseases should be especially vigilant in adopting preventive measures. A high-fiber diet, regular exercise, and maintaining a healthy weight become even more crucial in mitigating the genetic risk. Regular screenings

and check-ups can aid in the early detection of diverticulosis, allowing for timely interventions to prevent the progression to diverticulitis.

In summary, while genetics contributes to the risk of diverticular diseases, it interacts with modifiable lifestyle factors. A holistic approach to digestive health, considering both genetic predispositions and lifestyle choices, is key in managing and preventing diverticulosis and diverticulitis. Genetic research in this field continues to unveil new insights, offering potential avenues for targeted therapies and personalized interventions in the future.

Lifestyle Factors

Lifestyle factors play a pivotal role in the development and management of diverticular diseases, influencing both the onset of diverticulosis and the potential complications associated with diverticulitis.

Dietary Habits:
A low-fiber diet is a major contributing factor to diverticulosis. Insufficient fiber intake can lead to constipation and increased pressure in the colon

during bowel movements, facilitating the formation of diverticula. Conversely, a diet rich in fiber promotes regular bowel movements and helps maintain the health of the digestive system.

Physical Activity:
A sedentary lifestyle and lack of regular exercise are associated with an increased risk of diverticulosis. Physical activity aids in maintaining healthy bowel function and can reduce the likelihood of constipation, thereby mitigating pressure on the colon walls.

Obesity:
Being overweight or obese is a significant lifestyle factor that contributes to the risk of diverticular diseases. Excess weight can increase pressure within the colon, creating conditions conducive to the formation of diverticula. Adopting a healthy weight through balanced nutrition and regular exercise is essential for preventing and managing diverticular conditions.

Smoking:
Smoking is linked to an elevated risk of diverticulosis and diverticulitis. The harmful effects of smoking on blood vessels can compromise the blood supply to the colon, potentially contributing to the weakening of the colon walls.

Hydration:
Adequate hydration is crucial for maintaining digestive health. Insufficient fluid intake can lead to constipation, exacerbating the risk of diverticulosis. Staying well-hydrated supports smooth bowel movements and helps prevent the formation of diverticula.

Addressing these lifestyle factors through positive changes, such as adopting a high-fiber diet, engaging in regular physical activity, maintaining a healthy weight, quitting smoking, and staying hydrated, is instrumental in preventing diverticular diseases and promoting overall digestive well-being. These lifestyle modifications not only reduce the risk of diverticulosis but also contribute to the effective management of diverticulitis and its associated symptoms.

The Impact of Diet

Diet exerts a profound impact on the development, progression, and management of diverticular diseases, emphasizing the critical role of nutritional choices in maintaining digestive health.

High-Fiber Diet:
A diet rich in fiber stands as a cornerstone in preventing diverticulosis. Adequate fiber intake

promotes regular bowel movements, preventing constipation and reducing pressure on the colon walls. Whole grains, fruits, vegetables, and legumes are excellent sources of dietary fiber, contributing to the overall health of the digestive system.

Low-Fiber Diet:
Conversely, a low-fiber diet is strongly associated with an increased risk of diverticular diseases. Insufficient fiber intake can lead to constipation, forcing the colon to exert more pressure during bowel movements. This heightened pressure creates conditions conducive to the formation of diverticula. Reducing the consumption of processed foods and increasing fiber-rich foods can help mitigate this risk.

Hydration:
Adequate fluid intake is crucial for effective digestion. Proper hydration softens stool, aiding in its passage through the colon. Insufficient water intake can contribute to constipation, potentially exacerbating the risk of diverticulosis. Ensuring optimal hydration complements a high-fiber diet in supporting digestive health.

Impact on Diverticulitis Management:
For individuals with diverticulitis, dietary modifications play a key role in managing symptoms. A clear liquid or low-residue diet may be recommended during acute

episodes, gradually transitioning to a high-fiber diet as symptoms subside. Fiber supplements can also be beneficial in promoting regular bowel movements.

In essence, the impact of diet on diverticular diseases underscores the significance of making informed nutritional choices. Adopting a diet abundant in fiber, staying hydrated, and tailoring dietary habits to individual needs are pivotal steps in preventing and managing diverticulosis and diverticulitis, contributing to a healthier and more resilient digestive system.

Other Lifestyle Choices

Beyond diet, several other lifestyle choices significantly influence the risk and management of diverticular diseases, emphasizing the multifaceted nature of maintaining digestive health.

Physical Activity:
Regular exercise is crucial in promoting overall digestive well-being. Physical activity supports healthy bowel function, reducing the likelihood of constipation, a key factor in diverticulosis. Engaging in moderate-intensity exercises such as walking, jogging, or cycling can contribute to the prevention of diverticular diseases.

Smoking Cessation:
Smoking has been linked to an increased risk of diverticulosis and diverticulitis. The harmful effects of smoking on blood vessels can compromise the blood supply to the colon, potentially contributing to the weakening of the colon walls. Quitting smoking is a vital lifestyle choice to mitigate this risk.

Weight Management:
Maintaining a healthy weight is integral to preventing and managing diverticular diseases. Excess weight, particularly around the abdomen, increases pressure within the colon, fostering conditions conducive to the formation of diverticula. Adopting a balanced diet and regular exercise contribute to weight management and overall digestive health.

Stress Management:
Chronic stress can impact digestive function and exacerbate symptoms of diverticular diseases. Incorporating stress management techniques such as mindfulness, yoga, or meditation can positively influence gut health and support overall well-being.

Moderation in Alcohol Consumption:
While moderate alcohol consumption may not be directly linked to diverticular diseases, excessive alcohol intake can contribute to dehydration and

potentially exacerbate digestive issues. Maintaining moderation in alcohol consumption aligns with overall digestive health recommendations.

These lifestyle choices, when considered collectively, form a comprehensive approach to preventing and managing diverticular diseases. By incorporating regular physical activity, quitting smoking, managing stress, and maintaining a healthy weight, individuals can positively impact their digestive health and reduce the risk of diverticulosis and diverticulitis.

CHAPTER FOUR

Identifying Symptoms

Identifying symptoms of diverticular diseases, including diverticulosis and diverticulitis, is crucial for prompt diagnosis and effective management. While diverticulosis may be asymptomatic, diverticulitis often presents with noticeable signs.

Diverticulosis:
1. Asymptomatic: Most individuals with diverticulosis do not experience symptoms. The condition is often discovered incidentally during medical screenings or diagnostic procedures.

Diverticulitis:
1. Abdominal Pain: The hallmark symptom of diverticulitis is abdominal pain, usually on the left side. The pain can range from mild discomfort to severe and may persist for an extended period.

2. Fever and Chills: Inflammation of diverticula can lead to infection, causing systemic symptoms such as fever and chills.

3. Change in Bowel Habits: Diverticulitis can result in alterations in bowel habits, including constipation or diarrhea. Some individuals may also experience urgency or a feeling of incomplete bowel movements.

4. Nausea and Vomiting: In more severe cases, nausea and vomiting may occur, reflecting the systemic impact of diverticular inflammation.

5. Tenderness and Swelling: Palpable tenderness and abdominal swelling, particularly in the lower left abdomen, can be indicative of diverticulitis during a physical examination.

Prompt recognition of symptoms is crucial for seeking medical attention and initiating appropriate treatment. If symptoms such as persistent abdominal pain, fever, or changes in bowel habits arise, consulting a healthcare professional is essential for accurate diagnosis and the formulation of an effective management plan tailored to the specific presentation of diverticular diseases. Early intervention can prevent complications and contribute to the overall well-being of individuals with diverticulosis or diverticulitis.

Asymptomatic Diverticulosis

Asymptomatic diverticulosis is a common condition where small pouches, known as diverticula, form in the walls of the colon. The majority of individuals with diverticulosis do not experience any noticeable symptoms, making its presence often incidental and discovered during routine medical examinations or diagnostic procedures.

The lack of symptoms in asymptomatic diverticulosis stems from the fact that the diverticula themselves, while present, do not necessarily cause irritation or inflammation. These pouches may be detected during procedures such as colonoscopies or imaging studies conducted for unrelated reasons.

While asymptomatic diverticulosis generally does not require specific treatment, it underscores the importance of proactive measures for digestive health. Adopting a high-fiber diet, staying well-hydrated, and maintaining a healthy lifestyle can contribute to preventing the progression of diverticulosis and reducing the risk of complications.

It's crucial for individuals diagnosed with asymptomatic diverticulosis to stay vigilant about their digestive health, attending regular check-ups and screenings. Additionally, awareness of potential symptoms and prompt medical consultation if any arise can help manage the condition effectively and prevent the development of symptomatic diverticular diseases.

Importance of Routine Screening

Routine screening for diverticular diseases, particularly diverticulosis and diverticulitis, holds significant importance in proactive healthcare and disease prevention. While diverticulosis is often asymptomatic, routine screening methods can detect the presence of diverticula before symptoms manifest. Here are key reasons highlighting the importance of routine screening:

1. Early Detection:
Routine screenings, such as colonoscopies, can detect diverticulosis at an early stage, enabling timely intervention and preventive measures. Early detection allows healthcare providers to address the condition before it progresses or leads to complications.

2. Prevention of Complications:
Detecting diverticulosis early can help prevent complications such as diverticulitis, where the

diverticula become inflamed or infected. Timely management can reduce the risk of severe complications like abscess formation or perforation.

3. Symptom Recognition:

Screenings aid in recognizing symptoms associated with diverticular diseases, even when individuals are not actively experiencing discomfort. This facilitates a proactive approach to managing symptoms and preventing potential complications.

4. Personalized Health Plans:

Routine screenings enable healthcare providers to develop personalized health plans based on an individual's risk factors, health history, and the presence of diverticular diseases. Tailored interventions can include dietary recommendations, lifestyle modifications, and ongoing monitoring.

5. Improved Quality of Life:

Early detection and management through routine screening contribute to an improved quality of life for individuals with diverticulosis. Preventing complications and addressing symptoms promptly allow individuals to maintain optimal digestive health and overall well-being.

6. Population Health Impact:

Routine screening on a population level can contribute to the broader understanding of diverticular diseases, facilitating public health initiatives and awareness campaigns. Increased awareness encourages individuals to prioritize their digestive health and seek timely medical attention.

In conclusion, routine screening is a valuable tool in managing diverticular diseases by fostering early detection, preventing complications, and promoting overall digestive health. Incorporating routine screenings into healthcare practices supports proactive measures and enhances the well-being of individuals at risk for or diagnosed with diverticulosis.

CHAPTER FIVE

Symptoms of Diverticulitis

Diverticulitis, the inflammatory condition of the diverticula in the colon, presents with distinct symptoms that vary in severity. Recognizing these symptoms is crucial for timely medical intervention and management.

1. Abdominal Pain:
The hallmark symptom of diverticulitis is abdominal pain, often concentrated in the lower left side. The pain can be sudden, severe, and persistent, varying in intensity. In some cases, the pain may radiate to the back or the pelvis.

2. Fever and Chills:
Inflammation and infection of the diverticula can lead to systemic symptoms, including fever and chills. These signs indicate an inflammatory response and the presence of infection.

3. Change in Bowel Habits:

Diverticulitis can cause alterations in bowel habits, manifesting as constipation or diarrhea. Some individuals may experience urgency during bowel movements or a feeling of incomplete evacuation.

4. Nausea and Vomiting:

In more severe cases, diverticulitis may be accompanied by nausea and vomiting. These symptoms can result from the inflammatory response affecting the gastrointestinal tract.

5. Tenderness and Swelling:

Palpable tenderness, particularly in the lower left abdomen, is a common sign during physical examination. Abdominal swelling and bloating may also be observed.

6. Changes in Urination:

In some cases, diverticulitis can cause changes in urination, including increased frequency or discomfort. This is due to the proximity of the inflamed diverticula to the bladder.

7. Rectal Bleeding:

While less common, diverticulitis may lead to rectal bleeding. This can manifest as bright red blood in the stool or on toilet paper and indicates potential complications.

Prompt medical attention is essential if individuals experience these symptoms, as untreated diverticulitis can lead to complications such as abscess formation, perforation, or the development of fistulas. Seeking timely care allows for accurate diagnosis and the implementation of an appropriate treatment plan to alleviate symptoms and prevent complications.

Abdominal Pain and its Characteristics

Abdominal pain is a primary symptom associated with various digestive conditions, including diverticulitis. Understanding the characteristics of abdominal pain is crucial for diagnosing and managing underlying issues.

1. Location:
In diverticulitis, abdominal pain is commonly localized in the lower left side of the abdomen. This is a distinctive feature that often helps differentiate diverticulitis from other gastrointestinal conditions.

2. Sudden Onset:

The pain in diverticulitis can have a sudden onset and may intensify rapidly. Individuals may experience a sharp, cramping pain that can be severe.

3. Persistent Discomfort:
Unlike occasional discomfort, the pain associated with diverticulitis tends to be persistent and may last for an extended period. It can range from a constant ache to more acute pain.

4. Radiation:
In some cases, the pain from diverticulitis may radiate to the back or the pelvis, contributing to a broader area of discomfort.

5. Aggravation with Movement:
Certain movements, such as walking or coughing, may exacerbate the abdominal pain in diverticulitis. This characteristic can help healthcare providers in diagnosing the source of the pain.

6. Tenderness to Touch:
During a physical examination, the affected area of the abdomen may exhibit tenderness to touch. Palpating the lower left abdomen may elicit discomfort.

7. Associated Symptoms:
Abdominal pain in diverticulitis is often accompanied by other symptoms, such as fever, chills, changes in

bowel habits, nausea, vomiting, and abdominal swelling.

Recognizing the specific characteristics of abdominal pain associated with diverticulitis is essential for accurate diagnosis and effective management. Individuals experiencing persistent or severe abdominal pain, particularly with associated symptoms, should seek prompt medical attention for a comprehensive evaluation and appropriate intervention.

Changes in Bowel Habits

Changes in bowel habits are common symptoms associated with diverticulitis, highlighting disruptions in the digestive process. Understanding these changes is crucial for identifying and managing diverticular diseases.

1. Constipation:
Diverticulitis can lead to constipation, characterized by infrequent or difficult bowel movements. The inflammation and infection in the diverticula may alter the normal passage of stool through the colon.

2. Diarrhea:

Conversely, diverticulitis can cause episodes of diarrhea. Inflammation in the colon may result in an increased urgency to move the bowels and a looser stool consistency.

3. Alternating Bowel Habits:
Some individuals with diverticulitis may experience alternating patterns of constipation and diarrhea. These fluctuations in bowel habits can be disruptive and indicative of underlying digestive issues.

4. Urgency or Incomplete Evacuation:
Changes in bowel habits may also manifest as an increased urgency to have a bowel movement or a feeling of incomplete evacuation. These sensations can be attributed to inflammation affecting the normal functioning of the colon.

5. Blood in Stool:
In severe cases, diverticulitis may lead to rectal bleeding, presenting as bright red blood in the stool or on toilet paper. This symptom requires prompt medical attention.

Monitoring changes in bowel habits is essential for individuals at risk for or diagnosed with diverticulitis. Any persistent alterations, particularly when accompanied by abdominal pain, fever, or other concerning symptoms, warrant a thorough medical evaluation for accurate diagnosis and appropriate management.

CHAPTER SIX

Types and Severity of Diverticulitis

Diverticulitis can manifest in different types and varying degrees of severity, dictating the appropriate approach to management and treatment.

Types of Diverticulitis:

1. Simple Diverticulitis: This type involves localized inflammation and infection within the diverticula, typically without significant complications. It often presents with abdominal pain, fever, and changes in bowel habits.

2. Complicated Diverticulitis: As discussed earlier, complicated diverticulitis involves severe complications such as abscess formation, perforation, fistula formation, or obstruction.

Severity of Diverticulitis:

1. Mild or Uncomplicated: In mild cases, symptoms may include abdominal pain, usually in the lower left side, and mild systemic symptoms like fever and chills. The inflammation is confined to the diverticula without significant complications.

2. Moderate: Moderate diverticulitis may involve more pronounced symptoms, increased inflammation, and the presence of complications such as abscess formation. Medical intervention, including antibiotics and sometimes drainage, is typically required.

3. Severe: Severe diverticulitis often encompasses complications like perforation, significant abscesses, or fistula formation. Emergency medical attention is crucial, and surgical intervention may be necessary to address the complications and prevent further harm.

The severity and type of diverticulitis influence the choice of treatment. Mild cases may respond to conservative measures such as antibiotics and dietary changes, while severe or complicated cases may require hospitalization, more aggressive medical management, and sometimes surgery. Early recognition of symptoms and appropriate diagnostic evaluation are essential in determining the type and severity of diverticulitis, guiding healthcare providers in devising an optimal treatment plan for each individual case.

Uncomplicated vs. Complicated Diverticulitis

Diverticulitis, the inflammation of the diverticula in the colon, can be classified into two main categories: uncomplicated diverticulitis and complicated diverticulitis. Understanding the distinctions between these conditions is crucial for accurate diagnosis and appropriate management.

1. Uncomplicated Diverticulitis:
Uncomplicated diverticulitis refers to cases where inflammation is localized within the diverticula without the presence of severe complications. Common features include:
- **Abdominal Pain:** Individuals with uncomplicated diverticulitis typically experience abdominal pain, often concentrated in the lower left side. The pain may be sudden, severe, and persistent.

- Fever and Mild Symptoms: Fever and mild systemic symptoms such as chills may be present, reflecting the inflammatory response. However, these symptoms are generally less severe compared to complicated diverticulitis.

- Changes in Bowel Habits: Alterations in bowel habits, such as constipation or diarrhea, may occur.

2. Complicated Diverticulitis:

Complicated diverticulitis involves more severe complications and may include:

- Abscess Formation: In some cases, inflammation can lead to the development of abscesses, localized collections of infected fluid. Abscesses may cause persistent pain and require drainage.

- Perforation: Severe inflammation can lead to perforation of the diverticula, allowing the contents of the colon to spill into the abdominal cavity. This can result in peritonitis, a life-threatening condition.

- Fistula Formation: Complications may involve the formation of abnormal connections between the colon and adjacent structures, such as the bladder or other parts of the intestines.

- Obstruction: Inflammation and scarring may lead to partial or complete blockages in the colon, causing symptoms such as cramping, abdominal distension, and changes in bowel habits.

Treatment Approaches:

- Uncomplicated Diverticulitis: Treatment often involves antibiotics, dietary modifications, and symptom management. Hospitalization is usually not required unless symptoms are severe.

- Complicated Diverticulitis: Hospitalization, drainage of abscesses, and surgical intervention may be necessary to address severe complications.

In summary, distinguishing between uncomplicated and complicated diverticulitis is vital for tailoring appropriate treatment strategies. Uncomplicated cases often respond well to conservative measures, while complicated diverticulitis may require more intensive interventions, including surgical procedures. Early diagnosis and prompt medical attention are essential for optimizing outcomes and preventing potential complications associated with diverticulitis.

Differentiating Between Cases

Differentiating between cases of diverticulitis involves a comprehensive evaluation of symptoms, diagnostic findings, and potential complications. Here are key considerations in distinguishing between various presentations:

1. Symptom Assessment:

Uncomplicated Diverticulitis: Characterized by localized abdominal pain, changes in bowel habits, and mild systemic symptoms such as fever and chills.
Complicated Diverticulitis: Presents with more severe symptoms, potentially including persistent or escalating abdominal pain, fever, and signs of systemic illness.

2. Diagnostic Imaging:

Uncomplicated Diverticulitis: Typically diagnosed through imaging studies such as CT scans, revealing localized inflammation within the diverticula.
Complicated Diverticulitis: May show evidence of complications like abscesses, perforation, or fistulas, requiring more detailed imaging and assessment.

3. Physical Examination:

Uncomplicated Diverticulitis: Palpable tenderness in the lower left abdomen is common during physical examination.
Complicated Diverticulitis: Physical examination may reveal more pronounced tenderness, signs of peritonitis, or palpable masses associated with abscesses.

4. Severity Grading:

Mild or Uncomplicated: Limited symptoms and localized inflammation.

Moderate: More pronounced symptoms and potential complications.
Severe: Involves severe complications requiring urgent medical attention.

5. Response to Treatment:

Uncomplicated Diverticulitis: Typically responds well to conservative measures such as antibiotics and dietary modifications.
Complicated Diverticulitis: May necessitate more aggressive interventions, including drainage procedures, surgical consultation, or emergency surgery.

Clear differentiation between cases is critical for tailoring the appropriate management strategy. While uncomplicated cases often respond to conservative measures, complicated diverticulitis requires prompt and sometimes emergent interventions to address potential life-threatening complications. Early diagnosis, accurate assessment, and ongoing monitoring contribute to effective management and improved outcomes for individuals with diverticulitis.

CHAPTER SEVEN

Understanding Complications

Understanding the potential complications of diverticulitis is essential for healthcare providers and individuals alike. Complications can range from mild to severe, influencing the course of treatment and overall outcomes.

1. Abscess Formation:
In some cases, diverticulitis can lead to the development of abscesses—localized collections of infected fluid. Abscesses may cause persistent pain, fever, and require drainage procedures for resolution.

2. Perforation:
Severe inflammation can lead to the perforation of diverticula, allowing intestinal contents to spill into the abdominal cavity. Perforation can result in peritonitis, a serious and potentially life-threatening condition requiring urgent medical attention.

3. Fistula Formation:

Complications may involve the formation of abnormal connections (fistulas) between the colon and adjacent structures, such as the bladder or other parts of the intestines. Fistulas can lead to various symptoms and often necessitate specialized care.

4. Obstruction:

Inflammation and scarring may cause partial or complete blockages in the colon, resulting in symptoms like cramping, abdominal distension, and changes in bowel habits. Obstruction can require interventions such as surgery to alleviate.

5. Systemic Infections:

Severe diverticulitis can lead to systemic infections, with symptoms such as high fever, chills, and rapid heartbeat. Timely medical intervention is crucial to manage these complications.

6. Emergency Surgery:

In some cases, complications may require emergency surgical interventions, particularly in situations of perforation, extensive abscesses, or if other conservative measures prove ineffective.

Understanding these potential complications underscores the importance of early recognition and intervention. Prompt medical attention and tailored treatment plans are crucial to mitigate the impact of complications and improve the overall prognosis for individuals with diverticulitis. Regular monitoring, adherence to medical advice, and lifestyle modifications are essential components in managing and preventing complications associated with this gastrointestinal condition.

Grading Systems and Their Significance

Grading systems in diverticulitis provide a structured framework for healthcare professionals to assess the severity of the condition, determine appropriate interventions, and guide treatment decisions. Two commonly used grading systems are the Hinchey classification for complicated diverticulitis and the Ambrosetti criteria. Understanding these grading systems is vital for tailoring patient care.

1. Hinchey Classification:
This system categorizes diverticulitis into four stages based on the extent of complications:
- Stage I: Pericolic abscess
- Stage II: Pelvic, distant, or retroperitoneal abscess
- Stage III: Purulent peritonitis
- Stage IV: Fecal peritonitis

The Hinchey classification aids in determining the appropriate level of medical or surgical intervention, with higher stages indicating more severe complications.

2. Ambrosetti Criteria:
The Ambrosetti criteria assess the severity of acute diverticulitis based on radiological findings:
- Grade 0: Uncomplicated diverticulitis
- Grade 1: Pericolic air or small abscess
- Grade 2: Larger abscess, distant air, or free fluid
- Grade 3: Walled-off perforation
- Grade 4: Extraluminal gas or abscess

This grading system assists in stratifying diverticulitis cases and determining appropriate management strategies.

Significance:
Grading systems provide a common language for healthcare professionals to communicate the severity of diverticulitis, enabling consistent decision-making and facilitating effective collaboration among medical teams. The significance lies in guiding treatment approaches, predicting outcomes, and improving the overall management of diverticulitis based on the specific characteristics and complications associated with each case.

CHAPTER EIGHT

Treatment Options

The treatment of diverticulitis is multifaceted and depends on the severity of the condition, presence of complications, and individual patient factors. Here are key treatment options commonly employed:

1. Antibiotics:
For mild or uncomplicated cases, antibiotic therapy is often prescribed to control infection and inflammation within the diverticula. Commonly used antibiotics include ciprofloxacin, metronidazole, or amoxicillin-clavulanate.

2. Dietary Modifications:
A high-fiber diet is recommended for diverticulitis management. Increased fiber intake promotes regular bowel movements, reduces pressure in the colon, and aids in preventing future episodes. Fiber supplements may also be recommended.

3. Pain Management:

Over-the-counter pain relievers such as acetaminophen or nonsteroidal anti-inflammatory drugs (NSAIDs) can help alleviate abdominal pain. However, caution is advised with NSAIDs, as they may exacerbate symptoms in some individuals.

4. Hospitalization:

Severe or complicated cases may require hospitalization for closer monitoring, intravenous antibiotics, and potential interventions such as drainage of abscesses.

5. Surgical Interventions:

In cases of recurrent or severe diverticulitis, or when complications are present, surgical interventions may be considered. Procedures range from laparoscopic surgery to remove affected portions of the colon (sigmoidectomy) to more extensive surgeries in cases of complicated disease.

6. Lifestyle Changes:

Promoting a healthy lifestyle, including regular exercise, weight management, and smoking cessation, is crucial for preventing recurrent episodes and maintaining overall digestive health.

7. Individualized Care:

Treatment plans are highly individualized, taking into account factors such as age, overall health, and the specific characteristics of the diverticulitis presentation.

Effective management of diverticulitis often involves a combination of these treatment options, tailored to the unique needs of each patient. Regular follow-up with healthcare providers ensures ongoing evaluation and adjustment of the treatment plan based on the patient's response and any evolving aspects of the condition.

Antibiotics and Medications

Antibiotics play a pivotal role in the treatment of diverticulitis, particularly in managing the inflammatory and infectious aspects of the condition. The choice of antibiotics depends on the severity of diverticulitis and the presence of complications. Commonly prescribed antibiotics include:

1. Ciprofloxacin and Metronidazole:
This combination is often used for mild or uncomplicated cases of diverticulitis. Ciprofloxacin is effective against a broad spectrum of bacteria, while metronidazole targets anaerobic bacteria commonly associated with gastrointestinal infections.

2. Amoxicillin-Clavulanate:
This antibiotic is frequently prescribed for mild cases of diverticulitis. Amoxicillin, a penicillin derivative, is combined with clavulanate to enhance its effectiveness against a broader range of bacteria.

3. Augmentin:
A combination of amoxicillin and clavulanate, Augmentin is another antibiotic choice for managing diverticulitis, particularly when a broader antibiotic spectrum is necessary.

4. Individualized Antibiotic Therapy:
In more severe or complicated cases, healthcare providers may opt for different antibiotics based on the patient's health status, allergies, or previous antibiotic exposure.

While antibiotics are crucial for managing acute episodes, long-term use is generally not recommended. After the acute phase, dietary modifications, such as a high-fiber diet, and lifestyle changes are often emphasized to prevent recurrence. It's important for individuals to complete their antibiotic courses as prescribed, attend follow-up appointments, and communicate any adverse reactions or concerns to their healthcare providers to ensure the most effective and safe management of diverticulitis.

Role of Antibiotics in Diverticulitis

The role of antibiotics in diverticulitis is fundamental, primarily aimed at addressing the inflammatory and infectious components of the condition. Antibiotics play a crucial role in the management of diverticulitis by targeting bacterial overgrowth or infection within the diverticula, helping alleviate symptoms and preventing complications.

1. Controlling Infection:

In mild or uncomplicated cases of diverticulitis, antibiotics are prescribed to control and eliminate the bacterial infection associated with inflamed diverticula. Common antibiotics such as ciprofloxacin, metronidazole, or amoxicillin-clavulanate are effective in addressing the bacterial overgrowth.

2. Preventing Complications:

Antibiotics aid in preventing the progression of diverticulitis to more severe complications. By reducing the bacterial load and inflammation, antibiotics contribute to preventing the development of abscesses, perforation, or other serious complications.

3. Surgical Prophylaxis:

In cases where surgical intervention is needed, antibiotics may be administered before surgery to prevent postoperative infections. This prophylactic use is crucial in minimizing the risk of complications associated with surgical procedures.

4. Tailored Treatment:

The choice of antibiotics is often tailored to the specific characteristics of the infection, the patient's overall health, and any known allergies or sensitivities. This individualized approach ensures the most effective and safe antibiotic therapy for each patient.

5. Short-Term Use:

Antibiotics are generally prescribed for short durations to address the acute phase of diverticulitis. Prolonged or unnecessary antibiotic use is avoided to minimize the risk of antibiotic resistance and other potential side effects.

While antibiotics are a key component of diverticulitis treatment, they are often complemented by dietary modifications, lifestyle changes, and, in some cases, surgical interventions to provide comprehensive care for individuals with this gastrointestinal condition.

Other Medications for Symptom Management

In addition to antibiotics, other medications are often employed for symptom management in diverticulitis to address pain, discomfort, and associated gastrointestinal issues:

1. Analgesics:

Over-the-counter pain relievers like acetaminophen are commonly used to alleviate abdominal pain associated with diverticulitis. Nonsteroidal anti-inflammatory drugs (NSAIDs) are generally avoided due to their potential to worsen symptoms.

2. Antispasmodics:

For individuals experiencing abdominal cramping and spasms, antispasmodic medications such as dicyclomine may be prescribed. These drugs help relax the muscles in the intestines, reducing discomfort.

3. Bulk Laxatives or Stool Softeners:

In cases where constipation is a concern, bulk-forming laxatives or stool softeners containing fiber supplements may be recommended. These help maintain regular bowel movements and prevent straining during bowel movements.

4. Probiotics:
Probiotics, consisting of beneficial bacteria, may be suggested to promote a healthy balance of gut flora. While research on their efficacy for diverticulitis is ongoing, some individuals find relief from digestive symptoms with probiotic supplementation.

5. Prescription Pain Medications:
For severe pain that is not adequately controlled by over-the-counter options, healthcare providers may prescribe stronger pain medications. These are typically used on a short-term basis and require careful monitoring due to potential side effects.

6. Symptom-Specific Medications:
Depending on the individual's symptoms, specific medications such as anti-nausea drugs or medications to address changes in bowel habits may be prescribed to enhance overall symptom management.

It's crucial for individuals to communicate their symptoms effectively to healthcare providers, allowing for the development of a comprehensive treatment plan that addresses both the underlying inflammation with antibiotics and symptom relief with appropriate medications. As with any medical treatment, the use of medications should be closely monitored and guided by healthcare professionals.

CHAPTER NINE

Surgical Interventions

Surgical interventions for diverticulitis are reserved for cases with complications, recurrent episodes, or severe disease that does not respond to conservative measures. Here are key aspects of surgical interventions in diverticulitis:

1. Indications for Surgery:
- *Recurrent Episodes:* Individuals experiencing frequent or severe episodes of diverticulitis may opt for surgery to prevent further recurrence.
- *Complications:* Surgical intervention is often necessary when complications arise, such as abscess formation, perforation, fistula formation, or bowel obstruction.

2. Types of Surgical Procedures:

- *Sigmoid Colectomy:* The most common procedure involves removing the affected portion of the colon (sigmoid colon) where diverticula are prevalent.
- *Colostomy:* In severe cases, a colostomy may be performed, diverting the bowel through an opening in the abdominal wall. This may be temporary or permanent.
- *Laparoscopic Surgery:* Minimally invasive procedures, such as laparoscopic surgery, are increasingly utilized for certain cases, offering quicker recovery times and less postoperative pain.

3. Emergency vs. Elective Surgery:
- *Emergency Surgery:* In cases of acute complications like perforation or peritonitis, emergency surgery may be required.
- *Elective Surgery:* Elective surgery is planned for individuals with chronic, symptomatic diverticulitis or those at high risk for complications.

4. Risks and Benefits:
Surgical interventions carry inherent risks, including infection, bleeding, or complications related to anesthesia. The decision to undergo surgery involves weighing potential benefits against these risks.

5. Postoperative Care:
After surgery, patients require a period of recovery and postoperative care. Monitoring for complications,

managing pain, and gradually reintroducing a normal diet are essential components of postoperative care.

Surgical interventions in diverticulitis are carefully considered, and the choice of procedure depends on individual factors, the severity of the condition, and the goals of treatment. The decision to undergo surgery is typically made collaboratively between the patient and healthcare providers, considering the overall health and preferences of the individual.

When Surgery is Considered

Surgery for diverticulitis is considered in specific situations where conservative measures prove insufficient or when complications arise. Several scenarios prompt the consideration of surgery:

1. Recurrent or Severe Episodes:
Individuals experiencing recurrent and severe episodes of diverticulitis, despite adherence to conservative treatments, may opt for surgery to prevent ongoing flare-ups and improve quality of life.

2. Complications:
Complications such as abscess formation, perforation, fistula formation, or bowel obstruction often

necessitate surgical intervention. These complications pose significant risks and require prompt attention.

3. Unresponsive to Medical Management:
Cases of diverticulitis that do not respond adequately to antibiotics, dietary modifications, and other medical interventions may prompt consideration of surgical options.

4. Emergency Situations:
In emergency situations where there is acute perforation, peritonitis, or other life-threatening complications, emergency surgery may be unavoidable to address the immediate danger.

5. Chronic Symptoms Impacting Quality of Life:
For individuals with chronic symptoms significantly impacting their daily life, elective surgery might be considered to provide long-term relief and improve overall well-being.

6. Prevention of Future Complications:
Surgery may be considered in certain cases to prevent future complications, especially in individuals at a higher risk due to the severity or recurrence of their diverticulitis.

The decision to pursue surgery is highly individualized and requires careful consideration of the patient's overall health, preferences, and the specific characteristics of their diverticulitis. A collaborative approach involving open communication between the patient and healthcare providers is crucial in determining the most appropriate course of action for the management of diverticulitis.

Types of Surgical Procedures

Surgical procedures for diverticulitis aim to address complications, prevent recurrence, and improve overall quality of life. Several types of surgical interventions are employed based on the severity of the condition and individual patient factors:

1. Sigmoid Colectomy:
The most common surgical procedure for diverticulitis involves removing the affected portion of the colon, typically the sigmoid colon where diverticula are prevalent. This procedure, known as sigmoid colectomy, may be performed using traditional open surgery or minimally invasive laparoscopic techniques.

2. Colostomy:
In more severe cases, particularly when inflammation or complications are extensive, a colostomy may be considered. This involves creating an opening in the

abdominal wall, called a stoma, through which a portion of the colon is diverted. A colostomy can be temporary or permanent, depending on the individual case.

3. Laparoscopic Surgery:
Advancements in surgical techniques have led to increased utilization of laparoscopic or minimally invasive procedures. These involve smaller incisions, resulting in shorter recovery times, reduced postoperative pain, and improved cosmetic outcomes compared to traditional open surgery.

4. Bowel Resection:
In cases of severe complications or widespread disease, a more extensive bowel resection may be necessary. This involves removing a larger portion of the colon, sometimes including the affected sigmoid colon and adjacent segments.

5. Elective vs. Emergency Surgery:
Surgical interventions can be elective, planned in advance for individuals with chronic symptoms or recurrent diverticulitis, or emergency, required urgently for life-threatening complications like perforation or peritonitis.

The choice of surgical procedure depends on the individual patient's condition, the severity of diverticulitis, and the goals of treatment. The decision to undergo surgery is typically made through collaboration between the patient and healthcare professionals, taking into account the risks, benefits, and overall health considerations.

CHAPTER TEN

Dietary Guidelines for Management

Dietary guidelines for the management of diverticulitis are crucial for symptom control, preventing complications, and promoting overall digestive health. Here are key dietary recommendations:

1. High-Fiber Diet:
Emphasize a diet rich in fiber, including whole grains, legumes, fruits, and vegetables. Adequate fiber intake promotes regular bowel movements, softens stools, and reduces the risk of diverticula becoming irritated or infected.

2. Gradual Increase in Fiber:
For those not accustomed to a high-fiber diet, a gradual increase is advised to allow the digestive

system to adjust. Sudden changes may cause bloating or gas.

3. Hydration:
Maintain proper hydration by drinking an adequate amount of water throughout the day. Hydration helps soften stools and supports overall digestive health.

4. Probiotics:
Include probiotic-rich foods, such as yogurt with active cultures, or consider probiotic supplements to promote a healthy balance of gut bacteria.

5. Limiting Certain Foods:
While individual responses vary, some individuals find relief by limiting or avoiding specific trigger foods, such as nuts, seeds, and popcorn.

6. Low-Fat Diet:
Opt for a low-fat diet by reducing the intake of fried and processed foods. This supports overall gastrointestinal health and may reduce the risk of complications.

7. Regular Meal Patterns:
Establish regular meal patterns to promote consistent bowel habits. Eating smaller, more frequent meals may be beneficial for some individuals.

Individualized dietary plans, often developed in consultation with a registered dietitian, consider the patient's preferences, cultural factors, and any specific dietary restrictions. Adhering to these dietary guidelines forms a crucial component of the overall management strategy for diverticulitis, aiding in symptom control and supporting long-term digestive wellness.

The Role of Fiber

The role of fiber in the management of diverticulitis is paramount, contributing significantly to symptom relief and overall digestive health. Here are key aspects of the importance of fiber in diverticulitis management:

1. Bowel Regularity:
Dietary fiber plays a crucial role in promoting regular bowel movements. It adds bulk to stools, facilitating their smooth passage through the colon and preventing constipation.

2. Softening Stools:
Soluble fiber, found in foods like oats, beans, and fruits, absorbs water and helps soften stools. Soft stools are easier to pass, reducing the likelihood of diverticula becoming irritated or infected.

3. Prevention of Complications:

A high-fiber diet is associated with a lower risk of diverticulitis complications. Adequate fiber intake may reduce inflammation, lower the risk of diverticula becoming symptomatic, and prevent complications like abscess formation or perforation.

4. Gut Microbiota Balance:

Fiber serves as a prebiotic, nourishing beneficial gut bacteria. A balanced gut microbiota is essential for overall digestive health, supporting immune function and reducing inflammation.

5. Decreased Straining:

Fiber contributes to softer and bulkier stools, reducing the need for straining during bowel movements. Decreased straining minimizes pressure on the colon walls, potentially preventing the formation of new diverticula.

6. Prevention of Diverticulitis Recurrence:

For individuals with a history of diverticulitis, maintaining a high-fiber diet is associated with a reduced risk of recurrence. Fiber-rich foods contribute to a healthy colon environment, minimizing the likelihood of future flare-ups.

Emphasizing a diet rich in fiber, incorporating a variety of fruits, vegetables, whole grains, and legumes, is a fundamental component of diverticulitis management. It not only provides symptom relief but also supports long-term digestive wellness.

Recommended Daily Intake

The recommended daily intake of fiber varies based on factors such as age, sex, and individual health conditions. For adults, general guidelines suggest a daily intake of 25 grams for women and 38 grams for men. These recommendations, established by health organizations like the American Heart Association and the Academy of Nutrition and Dietetics, aim to promote optimal digestive health, prevent constipation, and reduce the risk of various chronic diseases.

It's important to note that these recommendations include both soluble and insoluble fiber, each offering unique health benefits. Soluble fiber, found in foods like oats, beans, and fruits, helps regulate blood sugar levels and lower cholesterol. Insoluble fiber, prevalent in whole grains, vegetables, and nuts, contributes to bowel regularity by adding bulk to stools.

Individuals with diverticulitis may benefit from a tailored approach to fiber intake. During periods of flare-ups, a low-fiber or a "low-residue" diet might be recommended temporarily to reduce strain on the digestive system. However, once symptoms subside, gradually reintroducing fiber-rich foods is crucial for long-term management and prevention of recurrence. Consulting with a healthcare professional or a registered dietitian can provide personalized guidance based on individual health needs and the specific challenges posed by diverticulitis.

Trigger Foods and Their Impact

Trigger foods can play a significant role in exacerbating symptoms for individuals with diverticulitis. While responses to specific foods can vary among individuals, certain items are commonly identified as potential triggers. Understanding and managing these triggers is crucial for symptom control and overall well-being.

1. Nuts and Seeds:
Whole nuts and seeds, due to their potential to get lodged in diverticula pouches, are often considered problematic. These foods may contribute to irritation or inflammation of the diverticula, leading to symptoms like abdominal pain.

2. Popcorn:
The hulls of popcorn kernels can be challenging to digest and may pose a risk of getting stuck in diverticula, potentially causing irritation and discomfort.

3. Certain Fruits and Vegetables:
While fruits and vegetables are essential for a healthy diet, some individuals may find that specific raw or fibrous varieties can trigger symptoms. For instance, citrus fruits or cruciferous vegetables might be problematic for certain individuals.

4. Spicy Foods:
Spicy foods may contribute to gastrointestinal irritation and increased bowel activity, potentially exacerbating symptoms such as abdominal pain and discomfort.

5. High-Fat Foods:
High-fat foods, particularly those that are fried or greasy, may be harder to digest and can lead to increased bowel movements, contributing to discomfort.

6. Dairy Products:
In some cases, dairy products may be challenging for individuals with lactose intolerance, potentially leading to gastrointestinal symptoms.

Identifying and avoiding trigger foods, often through a process of trial and error, can be crucial in managing diverticulitis symptoms. Consulting with a healthcare professional or a registered dietitian can provide personalized guidance, helping individuals develop a diet that minimizes triggers and supports optimal digestive health.

Portion Control Strategies

Effective portion control strategies are crucial for individuals managing diverticulitis, promoting digestive comfort and preventing symptoms. Here are key strategies to implement:

1. Use Smaller Plates:
Opt for smaller plates to create the visual illusion of a fuller plate. This can help control portion sizes and prevent overeating.

2. Listen to Hunger Cues:
Pay attention to hunger and fullness cues. Eating slowly and mindfully allows the body to signal when it's satisfied, reducing the risk of overconsumption.

3. Pre-portion Snacks:

Pre-portioning snacks into smaller containers helps prevent mindless snacking and promotes awareness of portion sizes.

4. Fill Half the Plate with Vegetables:
Prioritize vegetables, which are often low in calories and high in fiber. Filling half the plate with vegetables can help control overall calorie intake.

5. Use Measuring Tools:
Measuring cups and kitchen scales can provide accurate portion sizes, particularly for foods that may be more calorie-dense.

6. Share Larger Portions:
When dining out, consider sharing larger portions with a dining companion to avoid consuming excessive amounts of food.

7. Avoid Distractions:
Eating without distractions, such as television or smartphones, allows for better focus on portion sizes and internal hunger cues.

8. Be Mindful of Liquid Calories:
Consider the caloric content of beverages. Opting for water or other low-calorie options can contribute to overall portion control.

Implementing these portion control strategies can be beneficial for individuals with diverticulitis, helping manage symptoms and support overall digestive wellness. Tailoring these strategies to personal preferences and needs is essential for long-term success in maintaining a healthy and balanced diet.

CHAPTER ELEVEN

Lifestyle Modifications

Lifestyle modifications are integral to the effective management of diverticulitis, focusing on practices that promote digestive health, reduce symptoms, and prevent complications. Here are key lifestyle adjustments to consider:

1. Regular Exercise:
Incorporating regular physical activity supports overall health and aids in maintaining a healthy weight. Exercise can also contribute to optimal bowel function, reducing the risk of constipation.

2. Stress Management:
Chronic stress can impact digestive health. Stress management techniques, such as meditation, deep breathing exercises, or yoga, can help alleviate stress and potentially improve symptoms.

3. Adequate Hydration:

Proper hydration is essential for softening stools and preventing constipation. Individuals with diverticulitis should aim to maintain adequate fluid intake throughout the day.

4. Smoking Cessation:

Smoking has been associated with an increased risk of diverticulitis complications. Quitting smoking can have numerous health benefits, including a positive impact on digestive health.

5. Regular Bowel Habits:

Establishing regular bowel habits by maintaining consistent meal times and taking time for bathroom breaks can contribute to symptom control.

6. Avoidance of Trigger Foods:

Identifying and avoiding trigger foods that exacerbate symptoms is crucial. Lifestyle modifications may involve dietary adjustments to minimize the consumption of potential triggers.

7. Regular Check-ups:

Regular medical check-ups can help monitor the condition, identify any emerging issues, and ensure timely interventions.

8. Adequate Sleep:

Quality sleep is linked to overall well-being. Establishing good sleep hygiene practices can positively impact digestive health and immune function.

Lifestyle modifications, when integrated into a comprehensive management plan, can significantly improve the quality of life for individuals with diverticulitis. Consulting with healthcare professionals for personalized advice and guidance ensures that lifestyle adjustments align with individual needs and contribute to long-term well-being.

Hydration and Its Impact

Hydration plays a critical role in the management of diverticulitis, influencing various aspects of digestive health and overall well-being. Here's how adequate hydration impacts individuals with diverticulitis:

1. Softening Stools:

Proper hydration ensures that stools remain soft and easy to pass. This is particularly important for individuals with diverticulitis to prevent constipation and reduce the risk of diverticula becoming irritated or infected.

2. Bowel Regularity:

Hydration supports regular bowel movements, promoting a healthy digestive system. Consistent bowel habits help prevent complications and alleviate symptoms associated with diverticulitis.

3. Prevention of Dehydration:
Dehydration can exacerbate symptoms and contribute to complications. Maintaining adequate fluid intake helps prevent dehydration, supporting overall health.

4. Facilitating Nutrient Absorption:
A well-hydrated body enhances the absorption of nutrients from the digestive tract, ensuring individuals receive the necessary vitamins and minerals for optimal health.

5. Detoxification:
Adequate hydration aids in the detoxification process, helping to flush waste and toxins from the body. This can contribute to a healthier gastrointestinal environment.

6. Support for the Immune System:
Hydration is crucial for supporting the immune system. A well-hydrated body is better equipped to fend off infections and inflammation, which can be particularly important for individuals managing diverticulitis.

Incorporating sufficient fluids, primarily water, into daily routines is a fundamental component of diverticulitis management. Monitoring individual hydration needs and adjusting fluid intake based on factors like physical activity, climate, and health status ensures optimal digestive health and overall well-being.

Hydration Tips for Digestive Health

Maintaining optimal hydration is crucial for digestive health, especially for individuals managing conditions like diverticulitis. Here are essential hydration tips to support digestive well-being:

1. Consistent Water Intake:
Drink water consistently throughout the day. Sipping water at regular intervals helps maintain hydration levels and supports overall digestive function.

2. Monitor Urine Color:
Use urine color as a hydration indicator. Clear or light yellow urine generally suggests adequate hydration, while dark yellow or amber may indicate dehydration.

3. Hydrating Foods:
Include hydrating foods in your diet, such as fruits and vegetables with high water content. Water-rich foods

like watermelon, cucumbers, and oranges contribute to overall fluid intake.

4. Limit Dehydrating Beverages:
Reduce the consumption of dehydrating beverages like caffeinated and alcoholic drinks. These can contribute to fluid loss and may exacerbate symptoms in individuals with diverticulitis.

5. Hydration During Meals:
Consume water or other hydrating beverages with meals. This not only aids in digestion but also ensures you're meeting your fluid needs throughout the day.

6. Adjust for Physical Activity:
Increase fluid intake during periods of increased physical activity or in hot weather. Sweating can lead to additional fluid loss, emphasizing the importance of adequate hydration.

7. Set Hydration Goals:
Establish daily hydration goals based on individual needs, taking into account factors like age, weight, climate, and health conditions. This ensures a personalized approach to staying adequately hydrated.

8. Hydration Tracking:

Use apps or journals to track daily fluid intake. This helps maintain awareness and ensures that hydration goals are consistently met.

By incorporating these hydration tips into daily routines, individuals can actively support digestive health, reduce the risk of dehydration-related complications, and contribute to the overall management of conditions like diverticulitis.

CHAPTER TWELVE

Stress Management Techniques

Effective stress management is crucial for individuals with diverticulitis, as stress can exacerbate symptoms and impact overall well-being. Here are key stress management techniques tailored to support those managing diverticulitis:

1. Mindfulness Meditation:
Practicing mindfulness meditation involves focusing on the present moment, helping individuals cultivate a sense of calm and reduce stress levels. Mindfulness techniques can be integrated into daily routines to promote relaxation.

2. Deep Breathing Exercises:
Deep breathing exercises, such as diaphragmatic or belly breathing, can activate the body's relaxation response. These techniques help alleviate stress and tension, contributing to a more relaxed digestive state.

3. Yoga and Tai Chi:
Mind-body practices like yoga and tai chi combine gentle movements with focused breathing, promoting physical and mental well-being. These activities are known to reduce stress and improve overall flexibility.

4. Progressive Muscle Relaxation:
Progressive muscle relaxation involves tensing and then gradually releasing different muscle groups. This technique can help release physical tension and promote a sense of calm.

5. Regular Exercise:
In addition to its physical benefits, regular exercise is a powerful stress reducer. Engaging in activities like walking, jogging, or swimming can positively impact mood and overall stress levels.

6. Journaling:
Keeping a stress journal allows individuals to identify stressors and explore their emotions. This self-reflection can lead to better understanding and management of stress triggers.

7. Time Management:
Effectively managing time and setting realistic goals can reduce feelings of overwhelm, helping individuals navigate stress more effectively.

Adopting a combination of these stress management techniques empowers individuals with diverticulitis to cope with stressors, enhance overall well-being, and potentially reduce the impact of stress on digestive health. Integrating these practices into daily life supports a holistic approach to diverticulitis management.

The Gut-Brain Connection

The gut-brain connection is a complex and bidirectional communication system between the gastrointestinal tract and the brain. This intricate network involves neural, hormonal, and immune pathways, influencing both physical and mental well-being. For individuals managing diverticulitis, understanding the gut-brain connection is crucial as it can impact symptoms and overall health.

1. Influence on Digestive Function:
The brain and the gut communicate through the enteric nervous system, affecting various aspects of digestion. Stress or emotional factors can influence gut motility, potentially exacerbating symptoms like abdominal pain and discomfort in individuals with diverticulitis.

2. Impact on Immune Function:

The gut is a major component of the immune system, and the gut-brain connection plays a role in immune regulation. Stress and emotional states can influence immune function, potentially affecting the course of diverticulitis.

3. Stress and Inflammation:

Stress can trigger an inflammatory response in the gut, contributing to symptoms associated with diverticulitis. Chronic stress may exacerbate inflammation and potentially increase the risk of complications.

4. Role in Mental Health:

Conversely, the health of the gut can impact mental health. An imbalance in gut microbiota, often referred to as dysbiosis, has been linked to conditions like anxiety and depression.

5. Lifestyle Factors:

Factors such as diet, exercise, and sleep, which influence both gut health and stress levels, play a significant role in the gut-brain connection. Managing these lifestyle factors is essential for individuals with diverticulitis to support both digestive and mental well-being.

Understanding and addressing the intricate interplay between the gut and the brain is fundamental for individuals managing diverticulitis, emphasizing the importance of a holistic approach to health.

CHAPTER THIRTEEN

Long-Term Management and

Prevention

Long-term management and prevention are crucial aspects of diverticulitis care, aiming to minimize symptoms, reduce flare-ups, and prevent complications. Here are key strategies for individuals looking to manage diverticulitis over the long term:

1. Dietary Modifications:
Adopt a high-fiber diet rich in fruits, vegetables, and whole grains. Gradual introduction of fiber and monitoring trigger foods can help prevent constipation and minimize diverticulitis symptoms.

2. Hydration:
Maintain optimal hydration to support regular bowel movements and prevent dehydration-related

complications. Consistent water intake is particularly important for diverticulitis management.

3. Regular Exercise:

Incorporate regular physical activity into your routine. Exercise promotes overall health, aids in digestion, and helps manage stress, contributing to long-term diverticulitis management.

4. Stress Management:

Implement stress reduction techniques such as mindfulness, deep breathing, and regular exercise. Managing stress is crucial for preventing symptom exacerbation.

5. Medication Adherence:

For individuals prescribed medications, adherence to the prescribed regimen is essential. This may include antibiotics during flare-ups or medications to manage symptoms.

6. Routine Check-ups:

Schedule regular check-ups with healthcare professionals to monitor the condition, discuss symptoms, and address any emerging issues promptly.

7. Lifestyle Modifications:

Maintain a healthy lifestyle by avoiding smoking, limiting alcohol intake, and managing body weight.

These factors contribute to overall well-being and can positively impact diverticulitis management.

By adopting these strategies, individuals can actively participate in the long-term management and prevention of diverticulitis, promoting a balanced and healthy lifestyle that supports digestive health and reduces the risk of complications. Regular communication with healthcare professionals ensures that the management plan aligns with individual needs and health goals.

Part II. THE RECIPES

Living with diverticulosis/diverticulitis requires thoughtful consideration of dietary choices to manage symptoms and promote digestive health. While dietary recommendations may vary based on individual needs and the severity of symptoms, incorporating specific foods and preparation methods can contribute to a well-balanced and diverticulitis-friendly diet.

Diverticulosis involves the presence of small pouches, called diverticula, in the walls of the digestive tract, usually the colon. When these pouches become inflamed or infected, the condition is known as diverticulitis. While a high-fiber diet is often recommended to prevent diverticulosis, managing symptoms during flare-ups or in certain situations may involve temporarily reducing fiber intake and opting for easily digestible foods.

In this guide, we'll explore step-by-step processes for preparing various foods that align with dietary recommendations for diverticulosis/diverticulitis patients. From well-cooked vegetables and lean proteins to fermented foods and low-fiber options, these recipes and techniques aim to provide nourishment while minimizing discomfort.

It's important to note that individual responses to specific foods can vary, and consulting with a healthcare professional or a registered dietitian is crucial for personalized dietary advice. The recipes and guidelines presented here are intended to serve as general recommendations and starting points for those managing diverticulosis. As always, listen to your body, introduce new foods gradually, and make adjustments based on your own tolerance and preferences.

A diet for individuals with diverticulosis/diverticulitis typically focuses on promoting regular bowel movements, preventing constipation, and reducing the risk of complications. Here's a list of foods that are generally considered suitable for individuals with diverticulitis:

1. High-Fiber Foods:
  - Whole grains (brown rice, whole wheat bread, oats, quinoa)
   - Fruits (apples, pears, berries, bananas)
   - Vegetables (leafy greens, broccoli, carrots, squash)
   - Legumes (beans, lentils, chickpeas)

2. Lean Proteins:
   - Skinless poultry

- Fish
- Lean cuts of meat
- Plant-based proteins (tofu, tempeh, legumes)

3. Dairy:
   - Low-fat or fat-free dairy products (yogurt, milk, cheese)

4. Healthy Fats:
   - Olive oil
   - Avocado
   - Nuts and seeds (in moderation, depending on individual tolerance)

5. Fluids:
   - Water
   - Herbal teas
   - Broth-based soups

6. Probiotic-Rich Foods:
   - Yogurt with live cultures
   - Kefir
   - Fermented foods (kimchi, sauerkraut)

7. Cooked Vegetables:
   - Well-cooked vegetables may be easier to digest than raw ones.

8. Low-Fiber Foods (During Acute Episodes):

- In some cases, during acute diverticulitis episodes, a low-fiber diet may be recommended temporarily. This may include foods like white rice, white bread, and well-cooked vegetables.

It's important to note that individual responses to foods can vary, and what works for one person may not work for another. Additionally, recommendations may change based on individual symptoms and the presence of diverticulitis. Always consult with a healthcare professional or a registered dietitian to create a personalized plan tailored to your specific needs.

Moreover, some healthcare providers may recommend avoiding nuts and seeds, but recent research suggests that this advice might not apply to everyone with diverticulosis. It's crucial to discuss these recommendations with your healthcare provider and make dietary choices based on their guidance.

High-Fiber Foods

Steps to Making whole wheat bread

Making whole wheat bread for individuals with diverticulosis involves using whole grains, which can be a good source of dietary fiber. Here's a step-by-step process for making whole wheat bread:

Ingredients:

- 3 cups whole wheat flour
- 1 1/2 cups warm water (about 110°F or 43°C)
- 2 tablespoons honey or maple syrup
- 1 packet (2 1/4 teaspoons) active dry yeast
- 2 tablespoons olive oil or melted butter
- 1 teaspoon salt

Equipment:

- Mixing bowl
- Wooden spoon or electric mixer with a dough hook
- Plastic wrap or kitchen towel
- Bread pan
- Parchment paper (optional)
- Oven

Instructions:

1. Activate the Yeast:
   - In a small bowl, combine the warm water and honey (or maple syrup). Sprinkle the yeast over the water and let it sit for about 5-10 minutes until it becomes foamy. This indicates that the yeast is activated.

2. Combine Dry Ingredients:
   - In a large mixing bowl, combine the whole wheat flour and salt.

3. Mix Wet Ingredients:
   - Add the activated yeast mixture and olive oil (or melted butter) to the dry ingredients.

4. Knead the Dough:
   - Stir the ingredients together until a dough forms. Turn the dough onto a floured surface and knead for about 8-10 minutes until it becomes smooth and elastic. Alternatively, you can use an electric mixer with a dough hook for kneading.

5. First Rise:
   - Place the dough in a greased bowl, cover it with plastic wrap or a kitchen towel, and let it rise in a warm

place for about 1-1.5 hours, or until it has doubled in size.

6. Punch Down and Shape:
   - Once the dough has risen, punch it down to release the air. Turn it onto a floured surface, shape it into a loaf, and place it in a greased bread pan. Optionally, line the pan with parchment paper for easier removal.

7. Second Rise:
   - Cover the pan with plastic wrap or a kitchen towel and let the dough rise again for about 30-45 minutes.

8. Preheat the Oven:
   - Preheat your oven to 350°F (175°C).

9. Bake:
   - Bake the bread in the preheated oven for approximately 30-40 minutes, or until it sounds hollow when tapped on the bottom and has a golden-brown crust.

10. Cool:
    - Allow the bread to cool in the pan for a few minutes before transferring it to a wire rack to cool completely.

11. Slice and Serve:

- Once the bread has cooled, slice it into pieces and serve.

Remember to adjust the portion sizes and overall meal composition based on individual dietary preferences and tolerances.

Step-by-step process for preparing brown rice

Step-by-step process for preparing brown rice, a high-fiber whole grain suitable for many individuals, including those with diverticulosis:

Ingredients:

- Brown rice
- Water
- Salt (optional)

Equipment:

- Saucepan with a lid
- Fine-mesh strainer (optional)

Instructions:

1. Measure the Rice:

- Determine the amount of brown rice needed based on the number of servings. A common ratio is 1 cup of brown rice to 2 cups of water.

2. Rinse the Rice (Optional):
   - Rinsing the rice helps remove excess starch and can make it less sticky. Place the rice in a fine-mesh strainer and rinse under cold running water until the water runs clear.

3. Combine Rice and Water:
   - In a saucepan, combine the measured brown rice and water. Add a pinch of salt if desired. The salt is optional and can be omitted for those on a low-sodium diet.

4. Bring to a Boil:
   - Place the saucepan over high heat and bring the water to a boil. Stir the rice occasionally to prevent it from sticking to the bottom of the pan.

5. Simmer:
   - Once the water reaches a boil, reduce the heat to low to maintain a gentle simmer.

6. Cover and Cook:
   - Cover the saucepan with a tight-fitting lid to trap the steam. Allow the brown rice to simmer for about

40-50 minutes, or until the rice is tender and the water is absorbed.

7. Check for Doneness:
   - Around the 40-minute mark, start checking for doneness. The rice should be tender but still have a slight chewiness (al dente). If needed, continue cooking for an additional 5-10 minutes.

8. Fluff the Rice:
   - Once the rice is cooked, remove the saucepan from the heat and let it sit, covered, for a few minutes. Then, use a fork to fluff the rice gently.

9. Serve:
   - Serve the brown rice as a side dish or as a base for other dishes. It pairs well with vegetables, lean proteins, or legumes.

10. Store Leftovers:
   - If you have leftovers, store them in an airtight container in the refrigerator. Reheat as needed.

Remember to adjust the portion sizes and the overall meal composition based on individual dietary preferences and tolerances.

Step-by-step process for preparing Oats meal

Oats are a nutritious and fiber-rich option for individuals with diverticulosis. Here's a simple step-by-step process for making a basic bowl of oatmeal:

Ingredients:

- 1/2 cup old-fashioned oats
- 1 cup water or milk (dairy or plant-based)
- Optional toppings: fresh fruit, nuts, seeds, honey, or a splash of milk

Equipment:

- Saucepan
- Spoon

Instructions:

1. Measure Oats:
   - Measure 1/2 cup of old-fashioned oats. Adjust the quantity based on your dietary needs.

2. Choose Liquid:
   - Decide whether you want to use water or milk (dairy or plant-based). Both options are suitable for individuals with diverticulosis.

3. Combine Oats and Liquid:

- In a saucepan, combine the oats and the chosen liquid. If you prefer a creamier consistency, use milk.

4. Cook on Stovetop:
  - Place the saucepan over medium heat and bring the mixture to a simmer.

5. Stir Occasionally:
  - Stir the oats occasionally to prevent them from sticking to the bottom of the pan.

6. Cook to Desired Consistency:
  - Continue cooking until the oats reach your desired consistency. This usually takes about 5-10 minutes.

7. Optional Sweeteners:
  - If desired, add a natural sweetener such as honey or maple syrup. Keep added sugars in moderation.

8. Add Toppings:
  - Customize your oatmeal with healthy toppings like fresh fruit (e.g., berries, banana slices), nuts (e.g., almonds, walnuts), seeds (e.g., chia seeds, flaxseeds), or a splash of milk.

9. Serve:
  - Once the oatmeal is cooked to your liking and toppings are added, remove it from the heat and transfer it to a bowl.

10. Cool Slightly:
   - Allow the oatmeal to cool slightly before consuming.

11. Adjust Consistency:
   - If the oatmeal becomes too thick upon cooling, you can adjust the consistency by adding a little more liquid and stirring.

12. Enjoy:
   - Enjoy your bowl of oatmeal as a nutritious and fiber-rich breakfast or snack.

Remember that individual preferences may vary, so feel free to experiment with different toppings and flavors.

Step-by-step process for preparing Quinoa

Quinoa is a nutritious whole grain that can be a good choice for individuals with diverticulosis. Here's a step-by-step process for making quinoa:

Ingredients:

- 1 cup quinoa
- 2 cups water or vegetable broth

- Salt (optional)

Equipment:

- Fine-mesh strainer
- Saucepan with a lid
- Fork

Instructions:

1. Rinse the Quinoa:
   - Place the quinoa in a fine-mesh strainer and rinse it thoroughly under cold running water. Quinoa has a natural coating called saponin that can taste bitter, and rinsing helps remove it.

2. Combine Quinoa and Liquid:
   - In a saucepan, combine the rinsed quinoa and 2 cups of water or vegetable broth. If using water, you can add a pinch of salt for flavor (optional).

3. Bring to a Boil:
   - Place the saucepan over high heat and bring the quinoa and liquid to a boil.

4. Reduce Heat and Simmer:
   - Once boiling, reduce the heat to low, cover the saucepan with a lid, and let the quinoa simmer.

5. Cook Covered:
  - Allow the quinoa to cook covered for about 15 minutes. During this time, the quinoa will absorb the liquid and become tender.

6. Check for Doneness:
  - After 15 minutes, check the quinoa. The grains should be translucent, and you should see a tiny spiral (the germ) separating from and curling around each grain. If needed, continue cooking for an additional 5 minutes.

7. Fluff with a Fork:
  - Once the quinoa is cooked, remove the saucepan from heat. Use a fork to fluff the quinoa, separating the grains.

8. Let It Rest:
  - Let the quinoa rest, covered, for a few minutes to allow any remaining liquid to be absorbed.

9. Serve:
  - Serve the quinoa as a side dish or as a base for other meals. It pairs well with vegetables, proteins, or in salads.

10. Optional Additions:
  - Customize the quinoa by adding herbs, spices, or a squeeze of lemon or lime juice for additional flavor.

11. Store Leftovers:
   - Store any leftover quinoa in an airtight container in the refrigerator for future use.

Quinoa is a versatile grain, and you can incorporate it into various dishes to add nutritional value to your meals. As always, if you have specific dietary concerns related to diverticulosis, it's recommended to consult with a healthcare professional or a registered dietitian for personalized guidance.

Fruits

Step-by-step process for preparing Fruit

Preparing fruits for individuals with diverticulitis involves ensuring that they are easy to digest and gentle on the digestive system. Here's a general guide for preparing fruits such as apples, pears, berries, and bananas:

Wash and Peel (if Necessary):

1. Apples and Pears:
   - Wash the apples and pears thoroughly under running water.
   - Peel the skin if it's tough or if the individual prefers it peeled.

2. Berries:
   - Rinse berries (such as strawberries, blueberries, raspberries) gently under running water.
   - Remove any stems or leaves.

3. Bananas:
   - Peel bananas and discard the skin.

Cut into Manageable Pieces:

1. Apples and Pears:
   - Core the apples and pears, and then slice them into bite-sized pieces.
   - If slicing is challenging due to diverticulosis symptoms, consider cooking the apples or pears until they are soft.

2. Berries:
   - Berries are generally small and don't require cutting, but you can slice larger berries like strawberries if desired.

3. Bananas:
   - Slice bananas into rounds or mash them for a softer texture.

Cooking (Optional):

1. Apples and Pears:
   - If the individual prefers softer fruit or has difficulty with raw fruit, consider cooking apples or pears. You can sauté them in a bit of water or bake them until soft.

Combine Fruits:

1. Fruit Salad:

- Combine different fruits to create a fruit salad. Mix apples, pears, berries, and bananas for variety.
   - Add a squeeze of lemon juice to prevent browning if the fruit salad will be stored for some time.

Serving Suggestions:

1. Plain:
   - Serve the prepared fruits plain as a snack or a simple dessert.

2. With Yogurt:
   - Pair the fruits with plain yogurt for a nutritious and satisfying snack or breakfast.

3. Smoothies:
   - Blend the fruits into a smoothie with yogurt or a liquid of choice for a refreshing and easy-to-consume option.

Tips:

1. Moderation:
   - While fruits are generally healthy, moderation is key. Consuming a variety of fruits in smaller, more frequent portions may be easier on the digestive system.

2. Avoid Citrus if Sensitive:

- Some individuals with diverticulosis may be sensitive to citrus fruits. If so, consider limiting or avoiding citrus fruits like oranges or grapefruits.

3. Stay Hydrated:
   - Drink plenty of water, as the fiber in fruits can absorb water and aid in digestion.

Always consider individual preferences and tolerances when preparing fruits for someone with diverticulosis.

Legumes

Step-by-step process for preparing Beans

Preparing beans for individuals with diverticulitis involves careful cooking to make them more digestible. Here's a step-by-step process for making beans:

Ingredients:

- Dried beans (e.g., black beans, pinto beans, kidney beans)
- Water
- Salt (optional)
- Aromatics (optional, e.g., garlic, onions, bay leaves)

Equipment:

- Colander
- Saucepan or pressure cooker
- Wooden spoon

Instructions:

1. Select and Rinse:

- Choose the type of dried beans you prefer (e.g., black beans, pinto beans). Rinse the beans thoroughly under cold running water in a colander.

2. Soak (Optional):
   - Soaking beans overnight can help reduce cooking time and make them easier to digest. Place the rinsed beans in a large bowl, cover them with water, and let them soak for 8-12 hours.

3. Discard Soaking Water:
   - If you soaked the beans, discard the soaking water and rinse them again before cooking.

4. Combine with Fresh Water:
   - Place the beans in a saucepan or pressure cooker. Cover them with fresh water, using about 3 cups of water for every cup of dried beans.

5. Add Aromatics (Optional):
   - For added flavor, you can include aromatics like garlic, onions, or bay leaves. These can enhance the taste without adding excessive fiber.

6. Bring to a Boil:
   - If using a saucepan, bring the beans to a boil over high heat. If using a pressure cooker, follow the manufacturer's instructions for sealing and bringing it to pressure.

7. Reduce to Simmer:
   - Once boiling, reduce the heat to a simmer. Cover
the saucepan with a lid.

8. Cook Until Tender:
   - Simmer the beans until they are tender. The
cooking time can vary depending on the type of beans,
whether they were soaked, and the cooking method.
This can take anywhere from 45 minutes to 2 hours.

9. Add Salt (Optional):
   - Salt can be added toward the end of cooking, as
adding it earlier may toughen the beans. Taste and
adjust the seasoning if necessary.

10. Check for Doneness:
   - Beans are done when they are soft and easily
mashed between your fingers. Taste a few to ensure
they are cooked to your liking.

11. Serve or Store:
   - Once the beans are cooked, you can serve them as
is or incorporate them into various dishes.
Alternatively, store them in an airtight container in the
refrigerator for later use.

Tips:

- Start with Small Portions:
  Begin with small portions of beans to gauge tolerance and gradually increase as needed.

- Drink Plenty of Water:
  Ensure you stay hydrated, especially when consuming fiber-rich foods like beans.

- Consider Canned Beans:
  If cooking dried beans seems challenging, canned beans (rinsed and drained) can be a convenient and well-tolerated alternative.

Step-by-step process for preparing Chickpeas

Chickpeas, also known as garbanzo beans, are a good source of fiber and protein, making them a nutritious option for individuals with diverticulitis. Here's a step-by-step process for preparing chickpeas:

Ingredients:

- Dried chickpeas
- Water
- Salt (optional)
- Aromatics (optional, e.g., garlic, bay leaves)

Equipment:

- Colander
- Saucepan or pressure cooker
- Wooden spoon

Instructions:

1. Select and Rinse:
   - Choose dried chickpeas and rinse them thoroughly under cold running water in a colander.

2. Soak (Optional):
   - Soaking chickpeas overnight can help reduce cooking time and make them more digestible. Place the rinsed chickpeas in a large bowl, cover them with water, and let them soak for 8-12 hours.

3. Discard Soaking Water:
   - If you soaked the chickpeas, discard the soaking water and rinse them again before cooking.

4. Combine with Fresh Water:
   - Place the chickpeas in a saucepan or pressure cooker. Cover them with fresh water, using about 3 cups of water for every cup of dried chickpeas.

5. Add Aromatics (Optional):

- For added flavor, you can include aromatics like garlic, bay leaves, or onion. These can enhance the taste without adding excessive fiber.

6. Bring to a Boil:
   - If using a saucepan, bring the chickpeas to a boil over high heat. If using a pressure cooker, follow the manufacturer's instructions for sealing and bringing it to pressure.

7. Reduce to Simmer:
   - Once boiling, reduce the heat to a simmer. Cover the saucepan with a lid.

8. Cook Until Tender:
   - Simmer the chickpeas until they are tender. The cooking time can vary depending on whether they were soaked and the cooking method. This can take anywhere from 1 to 2 hours.

9. Add Salt (Optional):
   - Add salt toward the end of cooking, as adding it earlier may toughen the chickpeas. Taste and adjust the seasoning if necessary.

10. Check for Doneness:
   - Chickpeas are done when they are soft and easily mashed between your fingers. Taste a few to ensure they are cooked to your liking.

11. Serve or Store:
   - Once the chickpeas are cooked, you can serve them as is, use them in salads, soups, or other dishes. Alternatively, store them in an airtight container in the refrigerator for later use.

Tips:

- Start with Small Portions:
  Begin with small portions of chickpeas to gauge tolerance and gradually increase as needed.

- Drink Plenty of Water:
  Ensure you stay hydrated, especially when consuming fiber-rich foods like chickpeas.

- Consider Canned Chickpeas:
  If cooking dried chickpeas seems challenging, canned chickpeas (rinsed and drained) can be a convenient and well-tolerated alternative.

Lean Proteins

Step-by-step process for preparing Skinless poultry

Skinless poultry is a lean source of protein that can be included in the diet of individuals with diverticulitis. Here's a step-by-step process for preparing skinless poultry:

Ingredients:

- Skinless poultry (chicken breasts, turkey breasts)
- Olive oil or cooking spray
- Salt and pepper (optional)
- Herbs and spices (optional, for seasoning)

Equipment:

- Skillet or oven-safe pan
- Cooking thermometer (optional)

Instructions:

1. Select and Prep the Poultry:

- Choose skinless poultry cuts such as chicken breasts or turkey breasts. Ensure that they are trimmed of excess fat.

2. Season (Optional):
   - If desired, season the poultry with salt, pepper, and herbs or spices. Common choices include garlic powder, onion powder, paprika, thyme, or rosemary. Keep the seasoning simple to avoid excessive spice or fiber.

3. Preheat the Skillet:
   - Place a skillet or oven-safe pan on the stove over medium-high heat. Add a small amount of olive oil or use cooking spray to prevent sticking.

4. Cook in Skillet:
   - Place the seasoned poultry in the skillet. Cook until the underside is browned, typically 3-5 minutes, depending on the thickness of the poultry.

5. Flip and Cook the Other Side:
   - Flip the poultry using tongs or a spatula. Cook the other side until it's browned and the internal temperature reaches a safe level. The safe internal temperature for poultry is 165°F (74°C).

6. Check for Doneness:

- If using a cooking thermometer, insert it into the thickest part of the poultry to ensure it has reached the recommended internal temperature.

7. Oven Cooking (Optional):
   - If you prefer, you can transfer the skillet to a preheated oven (375°F or 190°C) to finish cooking until the poultry reaches the desired internal temperature.

8. Rest Before Serving:
   - Allow the poultry to rest for a few minutes before serving. This helps the juices redistribute and keeps the meat moist.

9. Serve:
   - Serve the cooked skinless poultry as the main dish. You can pair it with well-cooked vegetables, rice, or other diverticulosis-friendly sides.

Tips:

- Avoid High-Fat Cooking Methods:
   - Limit the use of frying or cooking methods that add excessive fat, as high-fat foods may be harder to digest.

- Use Lean Cuts:
   - Choose lean cuts of poultry, such as skinless chicken or turkey breasts, to reduce the fat content.

- Monitor Portion Sizes:
  - Be mindful of portion sizes to avoid overeating.

Step-by-step process for preparing Lean Meat

Lean cuts of meat can be a good source of protein for individuals with diverticulitis. Here's a step-by-step process for preparing lean cuts of meat:

Ingredients:

- Lean cuts of meat (e.g., sirloin steak, pork loin, lean ground beef, skinless poultry)
- Olive oil or cooking spray
- Salt and pepper (optional)
- Herbs and spices (optional, for seasoning)

Equipment:

- Skillet or grill
- Cooking thermometer (optional)

Instructions:

1. Select and Prep the Lean Meat:
   - Choose lean cuts of meat, such as sirloin steak, pork loin, lean ground beef, or skinless poultry. Trim visible fat to make the meat leaner.

2. Season (Optional):
   - If desired, season the lean meat with salt, pepper, and herbs or spices. Common choices include garlic powder, onion powder, paprika, thyme, or rosemary. Keep the seasoning simple to avoid excessive spice or fiber.

3. Preheat the Skillet or Grill:
   - If using a skillet, place it on the stove over medium-high heat. If using a grill, preheat it to a medium-high temperature.

4. Add Cooking Oil or Spray:
   - Add a small amount of olive oil to the skillet or use cooking spray to prevent sticking.

5. Cook in Skillet or Grill:
   - Place the seasoned lean meat on the skillet or grill. Cook until the underside is browned, adjusting the cooking time based on the thickness of the meat.

6. Flip and Cook the Other Side:
   - Flip the lean meat using tongs or a spatula. Cook the other side until it's browned and the internal temperature reaches a safe level. Use a cooking thermometer to check the internal temperature.

7. Check for Doneness:

- The safe internal temperatures for various lean meats are generally around 145°F (63°C) for beef, pork, veal, and lamb, and 165°F (74°C) for poultry.

8. Oven Cooking (Optional):
   - If you prefer, you can transfer the meat to a preheated oven (375°F or 190°C) to finish cooking until it reaches the desired internal temperature.

9. Rest Before Serving:
   - Allow the cooked lean meat to rest for a few minutes before serving. This helps retain juices and ensures the meat is tender.

10. Serve:
   - Serve the cooked lean meat as the main dish. Pair it with well-cooked vegetables, grains, or other diverticulosis-friendly sides.

Tips:

- Trim Visible Fat:
  - Remove visible fat from the lean meat to reduce overall fat content.

- Monitor Portion Sizes:
  - Be mindful of portion sizes to avoid overeating.

- Avoid High-Fat Cooking Methods:

- Limit the use of frying or cooking methods that add excessive fat, as high-fat foods may be harder to digest.

Step-by-step process for preparing Fish

Fish is often a well-tolerated protein source for individuals with diverticulitis. Here's a step-by-step process for preparing fish:

Ingredients:

- Fish fillets (e.g., salmon, tilapia, cod)
- Olive oil or cooking spray
- Lemon juice (optional)
- Herbs and spices (optional, for seasoning)
- Salt and pepper (optional)

Equipment:

- Skillet or oven-safe pan
- Baking sheet (if baking)
- Cooking thermometer (optional)

Instructions:

1. Select and Prep the Fish:
   - Choose lean fish fillets, such as salmon, tilapia, or cod. Ensure the fillets are fresh and free of bones.

2. Season (Optional):
   - If desired, season the fish with herbs, spices, salt, pepper, or a squeeze of lemon juice for added flavor. Keep the seasoning simple to avoid excessive spice or fiber.

3. Preheat the Skillet or Oven:
   - If using a skillet, place it on the stove over medium-high heat. If baking, preheat the oven to 375°F (190°C).

4. Add Cooking Oil or Spray:
   - Add a small amount of olive oil to the skillet or use cooking spray to prevent sticking.

5. Cook in Skillet or Bake:
   - Place the seasoned fish fillets in the skillet or on a baking sheet if baking. Cook until the fish is opaque and easily flakes with a fork. Cooking times can vary based on the thickness of the fillets.

6. Flip the Fish (if Using Skillet):
   - If cooking in a skillet, carefully flip the fish halfway through the cooking time to ensure even cooking on both sides.

7. Check for Doneness:

- Use a cooking thermometer to check the internal temperature of the fish. The safe internal temperature for fish is typically around 145°F (63°C).

8. Oven Broiling (Optional):
  - If baking, you can finish by broiling for a few minutes to add a golden crust to the top of the fish.

9. Rest Before Serving:
  - Allow the cooked fish to rest for a few minutes before serving. This helps retain moisture and ensures the fish is tender.

10. Serve:
  - Serve the cooked fish as the main dish. Pair it with well-cooked vegetables, grains, or other diverticulosis-friendly sides.

Tips:

- Choose Lean Fish:
  - Opt for lean fish varieties to minimize fat content.

- Use Cooking Techniques with Less Fat:
  - Consider grilling, baking, or broiling rather than frying to reduce the fat content.

- Monitor Portion Sizes:
  - Be mindful of portion sizes to avoid overeating.

Step-by-step process for preparing Plant-based proteins, including tofu, tempeh, and legumes

Plant-based proteins, including tofu, tempeh, and legumes, can be excellent choices for individuals with diverticulitis. Here's a step-by-step process for preparing plant-based proteins:

Tofu:

Ingredients:

- Firm tofu
- Olive oil or cooking spray
- Soy sauce or tamari (optional)
- Herbs and spices (optional, for seasoning)

Equipment:

- Skillet or non-stick pan
- Paper towels

Instructions:

1. Press the Tofu:
   - If using firm tofu, press it to remove excess water. Place the tofu block between layers of paper towels or

a clean kitchen towel, and press with a heavy object for about 15-30 minutes.

2. Cut into Cubes:
   - Once pressed, cut the tofu into cubes or slices, depending on your preference.

3. Season (Optional):
   - Season the tofu with herbs, spices, or a splash of soy sauce or tamari for added flavor.

4. Preheat the Skillet:
   - Place a skillet over medium-high heat and add a small amount of olive oil or use cooking spray.

5. Cook the Tofu:
   - Add the seasoned tofu to the skillet. Cook until the tofu is golden brown on all sides.

6. Serve:
   - Serve the cooked tofu as part of stir-fries, salads, or alongside vegetables and grains.

Tempeh:

Ingredients:

- Tempeh
- Olive oil or cooking spray

- Soy sauce or tamari (optional)
- Herbs and spices (optional, for seasoning)

Equipment:

- Skillet or non-stick pan

Instructions:

1. Slice or Cube Tempeh:
   - Slice or cube the tempeh into pieces suitable for your recipe.

2. Season (Optional):
   - Season the tempeh with herbs, spices, or a splash of soy sauce or tamari.

3. Preheat the Skillet:
   - Place a skillet over medium-high heat and add a small amount of olive oil or use cooking spray.

4. Cook the Tempeh:
   - Add the seasoned tempeh to the skillet. Cook until it's golden brown on all sides.

5. Serve:
   - Serve the cooked tempeh in salads, sandwiches, wraps, or as a protein addition to various dishes.

Legumes:

Ingredients:

- Dried or canned legumes (beans, lentils, chickpeas)
- Water
- Olive oil or cooking spray
- Herbs and spices (optional, for seasoning)

Equipment:

- Saucepan or pressure cooker (for dried legumes)
- Skillet or non-stick pan (for canned legumes)

Instructions:

For Dried Legumes:

1. Soak (Optional):
   - Soak dried legumes overnight to reduce cooking time. Rinse and drain before use.

2. Cook the Legumes:
   - Place the soaked legumes in a saucepan or pressure cooker, cover with water, and cook until tender. Cooking times vary depending on the type of legume.

For Canned Legumes:

1. Rinse and Drain:
   - Rinse canned legumes under cold water to remove excess sodium. Drain well.

2. Season (Optional):
   - Season the legumes with herbs and spices, or a splash of olive oil for added flavor.

3. Preheat the Skillet:
   - Place a skillet over medium heat and add a small amount of olive oil or use cooking spray.

4. Warm the Legumes:
   - Add the seasoned legumes to the skillet and warm them through.

5. Serve:
   - Serve the legumes as a side dish, in salads, or as a main protein source.

Tips:

- Experiment with Seasoning:
  - Play with different herbs and spices to add variety to your plant-based protein dishes.

- Combine with Vegetables and Grains:
  - Create balanced meals by combining plant-based proteins with well-cooked vegetables and whole grains.

- Stay Hydrated:
 - Ensure you drink enough water, especially when consuming fiber-rich plant-based proteins.

Dairy

Step-by-step process for preparing Low-fat or fat-free dairy products (yogurt, milk, cheese)

Low-fat or fat-free dairy products can be part of a diverticulitis-friendly diet. Here's a step-by-step process for incorporating these products into meals:

Yogurt:

Ingredients:

- Low-fat or fat-free yogurt
- Fresh fruits (optional)
- Honey or maple syrup (optional)

Instructions:

1. Choose Low-Fat Yogurt:
   - Opt for plain, low-fat, or fat-free yogurt. Check the label to ensure it doesn't contain added sugars or excessive additives.

2. Add Fresh Fruits (Optional):

- Enhance the flavor and nutritional value by adding fresh fruits like berries, sliced bananas, or diced apples.

3. Sweeten (Optional):
  - If desired, sweeten the yogurt with a drizzle of honey or maple syrup. Keep added sugars to a minimum.

4. Mix Well:
  - Mix the ingredients well to distribute the flavors evenly.

5. Serve:
  - Serve the yogurt as a snack, breakfast, or dessert.

Milk:

Ingredients:

- Low-fat or fat-free milk

Instructions:

1. Choose Low-Fat or Fat-Free Milk:
  - Select low-fat or fat-free milk to reduce the fat content.

2. Serve Cold or Warm:

- Enjoy the milk either cold or warm, depending on your preference.

3. Use in Recipes:
   - Use low-fat or fat-free milk in recipes that call for milk, such as smoothies, oatmeal, or soups.

Cheese:

Ingredients:

- Low-fat or fat-free cheese
- Whole-grain crackers (optional)
- Fresh vegetables (optional)

Instructions:

1. Choose Low-Fat or Fat-Free Cheese:
   - Select low-fat or fat-free cheese varieties. Consider options like part-skim mozzarella or reduced-fat cheddar.

2. Pair with Whole-Grain Crackers (Optional):
   - Enjoy the cheese with whole-grain crackers for added fiber and crunch.

3. Add Fresh Vegetables (Optional):
   - Enhance the snack by adding fresh vegetables like cherry tomatoes, cucumber slices, or carrot sticks.

4. Serve:
   - Serve the cheese as a snack or part of a light meal.

Tips:

- Check Labels:
  - When purchasing dairy products, check labels for added sugars and unnecessary additives.

- Moderation is Key:
  - Consume dairy products in moderation, especially if you have lactose intolerance. Choose lactose-free options if necessary.

- Stay Hydrated:
  - Maintain hydration by drinking water along with dairy products.

Healthy Fats

Step-by-step process for preparing Nuts and seeds

Nuts and seeds can be included in a diverticulitis-friendly diet in moderation, provided they are well-tolerated by the individual. Here's a step-by-step process for incorporating nuts and seeds into meals:

Nuts:

Ingredients:

- Nuts (e.g., almonds, walnuts, pecans)
- Fresh fruits (optional)
- Yogurt (optional)
- Honey or maple syrup (optional)

Instructions:

1. Choose Well-Tolerated Nuts:
   - Opt for nuts that are well-tolerated, such as almonds, walnuts, or pecans. Avoid nuts with added seasonings or excessive salt.

2. Portion Control:

- Practice portion control, as nuts are calorie-dense. A small handful (about 1 ounce) is typically a suitable serving.

3. Add Fresh Fruits (Optional):

- Enhance the flavor and nutritional value by adding fresh fruits like berries or sliced apple.

4. Combine with Yogurt (Optional):

- Pair nuts with low-fat or fat-free yogurt for a balanced snack.

5. Sweeten (Optional):

- If desired, sweeten the combination with a drizzle of honey or maple syrup. Keep added sugars to a minimum.

6. Serve:

- Serve the nuts as a snack, part of breakfast, or a topping for salads.

Seeds:

Ingredients:

- Seeds (e.g., chia seeds, flaxseeds, sunflower seeds)
- Yogurt (optional)
- Fresh fruits (optional)

- Honey or maple syrup (optional)

Instructions:

1. Choose Well-Tolerated Seeds:
   - Opt for well-tolerated seeds like chia seeds, flaxseeds, or sunflower seeds. Consider grinding flaxseeds for better digestion.

2. Portion Control:
   - Practice portion control, as seeds are also calorie-dense. A tablespoon or two is typically a suitable serving.

3. Combine with Yogurt (Optional):
   - Mix seeds with low-fat or fat-free yogurt for added texture and nutritional value.

4. Add Fresh Fruits (Optional):
   - Enhance the mixture by adding fresh fruits like berries or diced mango.

5. Sweeten (Optional):
   - If desired, sweeten the combination with a drizzle of honey or maple syrup.

6. Serve:
   - Serve the seed mixture as a topping for yogurt, part of a smoothie, or as an ingredient in oatmeal.

Tips:

- Chew Thoroughly:
  - Chew nuts and seeds thoroughly to aid in digestion.

- Stay Hydrated:
  - Drink plenty of water when consuming nuts and seeds, as they are rich in fiber and can absorb water.

- Monitor Tolerance:
  - Pay attention to your body's response and adjust portion sizes based on individual tolerance.

Step-by-step process for preparing Avocado

Avocado is a nutrient-dense and fiber-rich fruit that can be part of a diverticulosis-friendly diet. Here's a simple guide on incorporating avocado into your meals:

Ingredients:

- Ripe avocados
- Fresh lemon or lime juice (optional)
- Salt and pepper (optional)
- Whole-grain bread or crackers (optional)
- Fresh vegetables (optional)

Instructions:

1. Select Ripe Avocados:
   - Choose avocados that are slightly soft to the touch but not mushy. The skin should yield to gentle pressure.

2. Cut and Pit the Avocados:
   - Cut the avocado in half lengthwise, and twist the two halves to separate. Remove the pit by carefully tapping it with a knife and twisting.

3. Scoop Out the Flesh:
   - Use a spoon to scoop out the flesh of the avocado into a bowl.

4. Mash or Slice:
   - Depending on your preference, you can mash the avocado with a fork for a creamy texture or slice it into chunks for a chunkier consistency.

5. Season (Optional):
   - Add a squeeze of fresh lemon or lime juice to the avocado to enhance the flavor and prevent browning. You can also sprinkle with a pinch of salt and pepper if desired.

6. Serve on Whole-Grain Bread or Crackers (Optional):
   - Spread the mashed avocado on whole-grain bread or crackers for a simple and satisfying snack.

7. Pair with Fresh Vegetables (Optional):
   - Serve sliced or mashed avocado with fresh vegetables such as cherry tomatoes, cucumber, or bell pepper for added texture and nutrients.

8. Incorporate into Salads:
   - Add avocado slices or chunks to salads for a creamy and nutritious addition.

Tips:

- Control Portion Sizes:
   - Avocados are calorie-dense, so practice portion control. A recommended serving is typically about one-half to one whole avocado, depending on your dietary needs.

- Stay Hydrated:
   - Avocados contain fiber, so be sure to stay hydrated by drinking plenty of water.

- Monitor Tolerance:
   - Pay attention to how your body responds to avocado, as individual tolerance may vary.

- Include in a Balanced Diet:

- Incorporate avocados into a well-balanced diet that includes a variety of fruits, vegetables, lean proteins, and whole grains.

Fluid

Step-by-step process for preparing Herbal tea

Herbal teas can be a soothing and hydrating choice for individuals with diverticulosis. Here's a step-by-step guide on making herbal teas:

Ingredients:

- Herbal tea bags or loose herbal tea
- Hot water
- Optional: Fresh herbs or spices for flavor (e.g., mint, ginger)
- Optional: Honey or lemon for sweetness and flavor

Instructions:

1. Select Herbal Tea:
   - Choose herbal teas that are known for their mild and soothing properties. Examples include peppermint tea, chamomile tea, ginger tea, or rooibos tea.

2. Boil Water:
  - Boil water in a kettle or on the stove. Allow the water to come to a gentle boil and then let it cool slightly for a moment.

3. Prepare Tea Bag or Infuser:
  - If using tea bags, place one tea bag in a cup. If using loose tea, use an infuser or a strainer to contain the loose leaves.

4. Pour Hot Water:
  - Pour the hot water over the tea bag or loose tea leaves. Ensure the water is not boiling excessively to avoid scalding the tea leaves.

5. Steep the Tea:
  - Allow the tea to steep in the hot water. The recommended steeping time can vary depending on the type of herbal tea, but typically it's around 5 to 7 minutes.

6. Add Fresh Herbs or Spices (Optional):
  - Enhance the flavor by adding fresh herbs or spices. For example, you can add a sprig of fresh mint to peppermint tea or slices of fresh ginger to ginger tea.

7. Sweeten with Honey or Lemon (Optional):

- If desired, sweeten the tea with a teaspoon of honey or add a squeeze of fresh lemon for additional flavor. Be mindful of added sugars if you are watching your sugar intake.

8. Strain or Remove Tea Bag:
  - If using loose tea leaves, strain the tea to remove them. If using a tea bag, remove the bag from the cup.

9. Let it Cool Slightly:
  - Allow the tea to cool slightly before sipping to avoid burning your mouth.

10. Enjoy:
  - Sip the herbal tea slowly and enjoy its calming and soothing properties.

Tips:

- Stay Hydrated:
  - Herbal teas contribute to hydration, an essential aspect of digestive health. Ensure you drink enough fluids throughout the day.

- Experiment with Flavors:
  - Explore different herbal tea flavors to find the ones that are most appealing and soothing to you.

- Avoid Caffeine:

- Choose caffeine-free herbal teas, especially in the evening, to promote better sleep.

- Listen to Your Body:
 - Pay attention to how your body responds to different herbal teas and choose those that are well-tolerated.

Step-by-step process for preparing Broth-based soups

Broth-based soups can be a nutritious and well-tolerated option for individuals with diverticulosis. Here's a step-by-step process for making a simple broth-based soup:

Ingredients:

- Low-sodium vegetable or chicken broth
- Lean protein (e.g., chicken breast, turkey, tofu)
- Vegetables (e.g., carrots, celery, zucchini)
- Whole grains (optional, e.g., brown rice, quinoa)
- Herbs and spices (e.g., parsley, thyme, bay leaves)
- Salt and pepper to taste
- Olive oil (optional)

Equipment:

- Large pot

Instructions:

1. Prepare Ingredients:
   - Wash and chop vegetables, protein, and any other ingredients you plan to include in the soup.

2. Sauté Vegetables (Optional):
   - In a large pot, you can sauté aromatic vegetables like onions and garlic in a small amount of olive oil until they are softened and fragrant. This step is optional but can enhance the flavor of the soup.

3. Add Broth to Pot:
   - Pour low-sodium vegetable or chicken broth into the pot. Use enough broth to achieve the desired soup consistency.

4. Add Lean Protein:
   - If using chicken or turkey, add the lean protein to the broth. Simmer until the meat is cooked through. If using tofu, you can add it later in the process.

5. Add Vegetables:
   - Add chopped vegetables to the pot. Common choices include carrots, celery, zucchini, or any vegetables you prefer.

6. Add Whole Grains (Optional):
   - If desired, add whole grains such as brown rice or quinoa to the soup. Ensure they are well-cooked to aid digestion.

7. Season with Herbs and Spices:
   - Season the soup with herbs and spices. Common choices include parsley, thyme, bay leaves, salt, and pepper. Adjust the seasoning to taste.

8. Simmer Until Cooked:
   - Allow the soup to simmer until all ingredients are cooked and flavors meld together. The cooking time may vary, but it's typically around 20-30 minutes.

9. Adjust Consistency:
   - If the soup is too thick, you can add more broth to reach the desired consistency.

10. Remove Bay Leaves (if used):
   - If you added bay leaves for flavor, be sure to remove them before serving the soup.

11. Serve:
   - Ladle the soup into bowls and serve hot.

Tips:

- Start Simple:

  - Begin with a simple broth-based soup with easily digestible ingredients. As your tolerance improves, you can experiment with more ingredients.

- Hydrate Well:
  - Soups contribute to hydration, which is essential for digestive health. Drink plenty of water throughout the day.

- Monitor Portion Sizes:
  - Be mindful of portion sizes to avoid overeating.

- Avoid Excessive Fiber:
  - While vegetables and whole grains are nutritious, individuals with diverticulosis may want to start with smaller amounts and gradually increase fiber intake based on tolerance.

Probiotic-Rich Foods

Step-by-step process for preparing Yogurt

Making yogurt with live cultures at home is a simple process that can be a beneficial addition to the diet of individuals with diverticulosis. Here's a basic step-by-step guide:

Ingredients:

- Milk (whole, 2%, or skim, depending on preference)
- Yogurt starter with live cultures (store-bought plain yogurt with live cultures or a yogurt starter packet)
- Optional: Sweeteners or flavorings (e.g., honey, fruit, vanilla extract)

Equipment:

- Saucepan
- Thermometer
- Whisk
- Clean containers with lids for incubation
- Insulated cooler or warm environment for incubation
- Oven or yogurt maker (optional)

Instructions:

1. Heat the Milk:
   - Pour the desired amount of milk into a saucepan. Heat the milk gradually, stirring constantly, until it reaches about 180°F (82°C). This helps to denature the proteins in the milk.

2. Cool the Milk:
   - Allow the milk to cool to around 110°F (43°C). Use a thermometer to monitor the temperature.

3. Add Yogurt Starter:
   - In a small bowl, mix the yogurt starter with a small amount of the cooled milk. Whisk it until the starter is fully dissolved.

4. Combine Starter with Milk:
   - Pour the yogurt starter mixture back into the saucepan with the remaining cooled milk. Stir well to ensure even distribution of the starter.

5. Incubation:
   - Transfer the milk and starter mixture into clean containers with lids. Place the containers in an insulated cooler or another warm environment to maintain the temperature around 110°F (43°C) for the incubation period. This can take anywhere from 4 to 12 hours, depending on your desired thickness and taste.

The longer the incubation, the thicker and tangier the yogurt will be.

6. Check Consistency:
  - After the incubation period, check the consistency of the yogurt. It should have thickened, and you'll notice a tangy flavor.

7. Refrigerate:
  - Transfer the containers to the refrigerator and let the yogurt cool and set further. It's now ready to eat.

8. Optional: Flavor or Sweeten (After Cooling):
  - If desired, add sweeteners or flavorings such as honey, fruit, or vanilla extract after the yogurt has cooled. Mix well.

9. Serve:
  - Spoon the yogurt into bowls and enjoy it plain or as part of a meal or snack.

Tips:

- Use Quality Milk:
  - Choose high-quality milk, whether whole, 2%, or skim, based on your dietary preferences.

- Check Yogurt Starter:

- Ensure that the yogurt starter you use contains live cultures. You can use store-bought plain yogurt with live cultures as a starter for subsequent batches.

- Maintain Consistent Temperature:
  - During incubation, it's crucial to maintain a consistent temperature. An oven with a light on, a yogurt maker, or an insulated cooler can help with this.

- Experiment with Incubation Time:
  - The incubation time affects the thickness and taste of the yogurt. Experiment with different times to find what you prefer.

Step-by-step process for preparing kimchi and sauerkraut

Fermented foods like kimchi and sauerkraut can be beneficial for digestive health when consumed in moderation. Here's a step-by-step guide on making sauerkraut, a type of fermented cabbage, which can serve as a starting point for those with diverticulosis. Please note that individual tolerance to fermented foods may vary, and it's advisable to introduce them gradually into your diet.

Homemade Sauerkraut:

Ingredients:

- Cabbage (green or red)
- Salt (non-iodized, preferably sea salt or pickling salt)

Equipment:

- Large mixing bowl
- Clean quart-sized glass jar with lid
- Weight or cabbage leaves
- Clean cloth or paper towel

Instructions:

1. Select Fresh Cabbage:
   - Choose fresh, crisp cabbage. Remove any outer leaves that may be damaged.

2. Clean and Shred Cabbage:
   - Rinse the cabbage under cold water and remove any loose outer leaves. Shred the cabbage finely using a knife or a mandoline.

3. Add Salt:
   - In a large mixing bowl, combine the shredded cabbage with salt. The general ratio is about 1-1.5 tablespoons of salt per 2 pounds of cabbage. Use non-iodized salt to avoid interfering with the fermentation process.

4. Massage and Bruise Cabbage:
   - Massage and squeeze the cabbage with your hands for about 5-10 minutes. This process helps release the cabbage's natural juices.

5. Pack Cabbage into Jar:
   - Pack the cabbage into a clean glass jar, pressing it down as much as possible to submerge it in its own liquid. Leave some space at the top to avoid overflow during fermentation.

6. Use a Weight or Cabbage Leaves:
   - Place a weight on top of the cabbage to keep it submerged in the brine. Alternatively, use a couple of cabbage leaves as a cover.

7. Cover Jar:
   - Cover the jar with a clean cloth or paper towel, secured with a rubber band or string. This allows air to circulate while preventing debris from entering.

8. Fermentation:
   - Place the jar in a cool, dark place for fermentation. Check the sauerkraut every few days, pressing it down to ensure it remains submerged. The fermentation process typically takes 1 to 4 weeks, depending on taste preferences.

9. Taste Test:
   - Start tasting the sauerkraut after about a week to determine the level of fermentation you prefer. Once it reaches your desired taste, transfer it to the refrigerator to slow down the fermentation process.

10. Store in Refrigerator:
   - Store the sauerkraut in the refrigerator, where it can last for several months.

Tips:

- Maintain Cleanliness:
   - Ensure all equipment, including the jar and your hands, is thoroughly clean to avoid contamination.

- Experiment with Flavors:
   - Add other vegetables or spices to customize the flavor of your sauerkraut.

- Start Small:
   - If you're new to fermented foods, start with small amounts and gradually increase intake to gauge your tolerance.

- Consult a Professional:
   - If you have concerns about incorporating fermented foods into your diet due to diverticulosis or other

health conditions, consult with a healthcare professional or a registered dietitian.

This basic process can also be adapted for making kimchi or other fermented vegetables. Always listen to your body and consult with healthcare professionals for personalized dietary advice.

Cooked Vegetables

Step-by-step process for preparing Vegetables

Well-cooked vegetables can be easier on the digestive system for individuals with diverticulosis. Here's a step-by-step process for making well-cooked vegetables:

Ingredients:

- Vegetables of choice (e.g., carrots, zucchini, spinach, bell peppers)
- Olive oil or a low-fat cooking spray
- Herbs and spices for seasoning (optional)
- Salt and pepper to taste

Equipment:

- Cutting board
- Knife
- Steamer or saucepan with lid
- Skillet or non-stick pan (optional)

Instructions:

1. Select Vegetables:

   - Choose easily digestible vegetables such as carrots, zucchini, or spinach. Avoid raw vegetables or those with tough fibers.

2. Wash and Prep:
   - Wash the vegetables thoroughly. Peel and chop them into bite-sized pieces.

3. Steam or Boil:
   - Use a steamer or a saucepan with a lid to steam or boil the vegetables. Steaming is preferable as it retains more nutrients. If boiling, ensure not to overcook, as this can lead to mushiness.

4. Check Doneness:
   - Test the vegetables for doneness by inserting a fork or knife. They should be tender but not overly soft.

5. Sauté (Optional):
   - For added flavor, you can sauté the steamed or boiled vegetables in a skillet. Use a small amount of olive oil or a low-fat cooking spray. Season with herbs and spices if desired.

6. Season:
   - Season the vegetables with a pinch of salt and pepper. You can also add herbs like thyme, rosemary, or a squeeze of lemon for additional flavor.

7. Serve Warm:
  - Serve the well-cooked vegetables warm as a side dish or part of a meal.

Tips:

- Choose Well-Tolerated Vegetables:
  - Opt for vegetables that are well-tolerated and do not cause discomfort. Experiment with different vegetables to find those that suit you.

- Avoid Overcooking:
  - Overcooking vegetables can lead to nutrient loss and a less appealing texture. Cook until they are tender but still retain some firmness.

- Use Gentle Cooking Methods:
  - Steaming and sautéing with minimal oil are gentle cooking methods that help preserve the nutritional content of vegetables.

- Monitor Fiber Intake:
  - While well-cooked vegetables are easier to digest, it's essential to monitor your overall fiber intake. Gradually introduce fiber-rich foods and adjust based on your tolerance.

- Stay Hydrated:

- Ensure you stay hydrated, especially when consuming fiber-rich foods.

Always consult with a healthcare professional or a registered dietitian for personalized dietary advice, especially if you have specific concerns or restrictions related to diverticulosis.

Low-Fiber Foods

Step-by-step process for preparing

Low-fiber foods can be recommended for individuals with diverticulosis during certain phases or flare-ups. Here's a step-by-step process for making a simple meal featuring low-fiber foods:

Low-Fiber Chicken and Rice Dish:

Ingredients:

- Boneless, skinless chicken breast or thighs
- White rice or refined grains
- Low-fiber vegetables (e.g., peeled and cooked carrots, well-cooked zucchini)
- Olive oil or low-fat cooking spray
- Salt, pepper, and mild herbs or spices for seasoning

Equipment:

- Skillet or non-stick pan
- Saucepan for cooking rice
- Cutting board
- Knife

Instructions:

1. Prepare Chicken:
   - Trim any excess fat from the chicken breast or thighs. Season with a small amount of salt, pepper, and mild herbs or spices of your choice.

2. Cook Chicken:
   - In a skillet over medium heat, add a small amount of olive oil or use a low-fat cooking spray. Cook the chicken until it's fully cooked and reaches a safe internal temperature (165°F or 74°C).

3. Prepare Rice:
   - While the chicken is cooking, prepare white rice or another refined grain according to the package instructions. White rice is generally lower in fiber than brown rice.

4. Cook Low-Fiber Vegetables:
   - Choose low-fiber vegetables that have been peeled and are well-cooked, such as carrots or zucchini. Sauté them in the skillet with a small amount of oil until they are tender.

5. Combine Ingredients:

- Once the chicken, rice, and vegetables are cooked, combine them in the skillet. Mix gently to incorporate the flavors.

6. Season to Taste:
  - Season the dish with additional salt, pepper, or mild herbs and spices to taste.

7. Serve Warm:
  - Plate the low-fiber chicken and rice dish and serve it warm.

Tips:

- Choose Refined Grains:
  - Opt for refined grains like white rice during periods when low-fiber foods are recommended.

- Select Well-Cooked Vegetables:
  - Choose vegetables that are well-cooked and peeled, such as carrots or zucchini, to reduce fiber content.

- Monitor Portion Sizes:
  - Be mindful of portion sizes to avoid overeating. Eating smaller, more frequent meals may be beneficial.

- Stay Hydrated:
  - Ensure you stay hydrated, especially when consuming lower-fiber foods.

- Gradually Reintroduce Fiber:
 - As your symptoms improve, you can gradually reintroduce higher-fiber foods back into your diet. Consult with a healthcare professional or dietitian for personalized guidance.

It's crucial to note that a low-fiber diet should be temporary, and it's important to reintroduce fiber gradually for long-term digestive health.